the
PCOS
Health & Nutrition Guide

Includes **125** Recipes for Managing Polycystic Ovarian Syndrome

Dr. Jillian Stansbury, ND
with Dr. Sheila Mitchell, MD

Robert
ROSE

For complete cataloguing information, see page 281.

Disclaimer

This book is a general guide only and should never be a substitute for the skill, knowledge, and experience of a qualified medical professional dealing with the facts, circumstances, and symptoms of a particular case.

The nutritional, medical, and health information presented in this book is based on the research, training, and professional experience of the author, and is true and complete to the best of her knowledge. However, this book is intended only as an informative guide for those wishing to know more about health, nutrition, and medicine; it is not intended to replace or countermand the advice given by the reader's personal physician. Because each person and situation is unique, the author and the publisher urge the reader to check with a qualified health-care professional before using any procedure where there is a question as to its appropriateness. A physician should be consulted before beginning any exercise program. The author and the publisher are not responsible for any adverse effects or consequences resulting from the use of the information in this book. It is the responsibility of the reader to consult a physician or other qualified health-care professional regarding his or her personal care.

This book contains references to products that may not be available everywhere. The intent of the information provided is to be helpful; however, there is no guarantee of results associated with the information provided. Use of brand names is for educational purposes only and does not imply endorsement.

The recipes in this book have been carefully tested by our kitchen and our tasters. To the best of our knowledge, they are safe and nutritious for ordinary use and users. For those people with food or other allergies, or who have special food requirements or health issues, please read the suggested contents of each recipe carefully and determine whether or not they may create a problem for you. All recipes are used at the risk of the consumer. We cannot be responsible for any hazards, loss or damage that may occur as a result of any recipe use. For those with special needs, allergies, requirements or health problems, in the event of any doubt, please contact your medical adviser prior to the use of any recipe.

Design and Production: Daniella Zanchetta/PageWave Graphics Inc.
Editor: Bob Hilderley, Senior Editor, Health
Copyeditor: Kelly Jones
Proofreader: Sheila Wawanash
Indexer: Gillian Watts
Illustrations: Guy Parsons/Three in a Box
Cover image: © Ekely/iStockphoto.com

We acknowledge the financial support of the Government of Canada through the Book Publishing Industry Development Program (BPIDP) for our publishing activities.

Published by Robert Rose Inc.
120 Eglinton Avenue East, Suite 800, Toronto, Ontario, Canada M4P 1E2
Tel: (416) 322-6552 Fax: (416) 322-6936
www.robertrose.ca

Printed and bound in Canada

1 2 3 4 5 6 7 8 9 MP 20 19 18 17 16 15 14 13 12

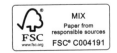

Contents

Quick Guide *to* PCOS Diet and Supplements

PCOS Dietary Program

- High complex carbohydrate foods
- Low glycemic index foods
- Whole foods
- High-fiber foods
- High-protein foods
- High essential fatty acid foods
- Therapeutic superfoods

PCOS Superfoods

- Flaxseed
- Legumes
- Sprouted legumes and grains
- Buckwheat
- Brewer's yeast
- Maca powder
- Nut meal and milks
- Organic foods

PCOS Therapeutic Nutrients

- Vitamin D
- Chromium
- N-acetylcysteine (NAC)
- B vitamins
- *D-chiro-inositol* and *pinitol*
- Lecithin
- Antioxidants
- Magnesium

PCOS Medicinal Herbs

- *Opuntia ficus-indica* (prickly pear cactus)
- *Stevia rebaudiana* (stevia)
- *Lepidium meyenii* (maca)
- *Pueraria tuberosa* (pueraria, Indian kudzu)
- *Astragalus membranaceus* (milkvetch)
- *Medicago sativa* (alfalfa)
- *Glycyrrhiza glabra* (licorice)
- *Trigonella foenum-graceum* (fenugreek)
- *Vaccinium* species (blueberries, bilberries)
- *Mahonia aquifolium* (Oregon grape)
- *Hydrastis canadensis* (goldenseal)
- *Silybum marianum* (milk thistle)
- *Vitex agnus-castus* (chaste tree berry)
- *Serenoa repens* (saw palmetto)
- *Commiphora mukul* (guggul)
- *Ginkgo biloba* (maidenhair tree)
- *Allium cepa* (onions)
- *Allium sativum* (garlic)
- *Hibiscus sabdariffa* (hibiscus)
- *Oenothera biennis* (evening primrose)
- *Ribes* species (currant seed)
- *Linum ussitatissimum* (flaxseed)

Introduction

❧ *Heidi*

Heidi, a pretty blond with an easy smile, sat across from me in my book-filled consultation room and described why she had come to see me. "My husband and I have been trying to get pregnant for almost a year, but so far no luck," she told me. "I went to my doctor, who I've been going to since I was a kid, and he gave me a physical and ran some blood work." She handed me the papers. "He told me everything was fine. I thought I'd see if you had any ideas."

I glanced at the papers immediately. I thought her glucose was too high at 107, although it was not so high as to be considered above the normal range. Her cholesterol was 207, just a few points above the upper limit of normal, and all the other test results fell within the normal limits. As I spoke with Heidi over the next hour, I became suspicious that she had a complex hormonal imbalance called polycystic ovarian syndrome, or PCOS. I was concerned for Heidi not only because of the emotional and physical hardships she might suffer in trying to have a child, but because the hormonal imbalances also put her at risk for reproductive cancers, heart disease, and diabetes.

During our first visit, Heidi detailed her irregular menstrual cycles, her struggle with her weight, and her months of electrolysis to get rid of her "peach fuzz" blond moustache. Heidi's mother was diabetic, and both of her parents were on medications to control their high cholesterol and blood pressure. I was worried that — given another decade — this would be Heidi's fate as well if something was not done immediately to correct the hormonal and metabolic imbalances. Heidi was seeking help for her infertility, and I saw this as an opportunity to prevent her from becoming diabetic, developing heart disease, or, worse, developing ovarian or another reproductive cancer down the road.

Heidi and I began by focusing on her diet and nutrition. PCOS may be associated with an inability of the body's cells to respond to insulin, a hormone from the pancreas that helps sugar in the blood move into the cells. Diet and nutrition can help improve the cells' response to insulin. I prescribed a specific diet and recommended several nutritional supplements.

Heidi's diet was devised to lower her blood sugar level and improve her insulin response, using foods she liked well enough to stick with the diet. We cut down on the breads and carbs and ramped up the salads and vegetables. We got rid of the sugar and soda pop altogether, and we worked out a long list of bean dishes with enough diversity to have a different legume every day of the week.

PCOS is also associated with elevated androgens, the so-called male hormones. Heidi's facial hair was likely related to excess testosterone, and lab testing confirmed the suspicion. Elevated testosterone also interferes with fertility, so we worked with herbal therapies to help balance her hormones. Heidi's menstrual cycles, which had been somewhat irregular, became more or less monthly and predictable — a boon when trying to conceive.

Once her blood sugar and hormonal balance improved, about 8 months after her first visit, we began fertility support therapies in earnest, turning our attention to enhancing ovulation, improving circulation in the uterus, and ingesting fertility-supporting herbs and nutrients. Heidi conceived 3 months later, and gave birth to a healthy girl.

Although the name Heidi is a pseudonym, this is a true story — and hers is similar to many of the stories I hear from women of all ages visiting my small-town practice in Washington State and from my colleagues at the National College of Natural Medicine, where I am an associate professor of botanical medicine.

Polycystic ovarian syndrome (PCOS) is a complex hormonal disorder characterized by insulin resistance, elevated androgens, and thyroid dysfunction. In 50% of cases, cysts develop on the ovaries. This condition can cause menstrual irregularities and infertility. PCOS has many other serious consequences beyond fertility and menstrual problems. Women with PCOS are at increased risk for diabetes, chronic obesity, heart disease, thyroid disorders, and hormonal cancers. The most common treatments for PCOS are dietary therapy, nutritional supplements, and medicinal herbs, which can help restore hormonal balance and decrease the risk of developing these associated conditions.

The presentation of PCOS can be so subtle that it is missed by many physicians, but this problem is being dispelled by the increasing amount of evidence-based PCOS research appearing in respected medical journals. This book would not be possible without that body of research, which underpins everything we recommend.

This book provides the information all women need to know about the cause and progression of PCOS, and sets out a plan to prevent this condition and treat it effectively if you already have PCOS. This is one condition you can become actively involved in resolving.

Part 1

Understanding PCOS

Chapter 1

What Is PCOS?

CASE HISTORY
❧ *Margaret*

When she first came to our clinic to learn more about her recent diagnosis of diabetes, Margaret was a fleshy, round-faced, 55-year-old secretary weighing more than 200 pounds (90 kg). Given her five foot two frame, she was considered obese. She was currently postmenopausal, but she reported a long history of irregular menses, PMS, and significant acne from which she still bore the scars. Margaret and her husband had tried for many years to become pregnant but never succeeded, even with two expensive in vitro fertilization attempts. No one had diagnosed her as having PCOS, yet the evidence was glaring.

Her occasional physical exams and visits to her primary physician always resulted in a lecture to lose some weight, and 2 weeks after her appointments she would receive a postcard from her doctor reminding her that her cholesterol and blood glucose were a "little too high" with no comment on how to go about making any changes. She tried to lose weight by choosing "low fat" foods, but she would get nowhere. Her most recent physical was followed by a postcard with the message "Blood sugar in the diabetic range. Please schedule a follow-up appointment."

The treatment Margaret and I undertook was extensive and multipronged, encompassing many of the ideas presented in this book. The key therapies, however, might be our dietary efforts. Margaret thought eating toast with no butter was doing the right thing because it eliminated the fat. She did not realize that her high cholesterol was as much related to her carbohydrate intake as it was to the fat intake. She chose low-fat pretzels over chips and whole-grain bagels over the doughnuts she really wanted. Margaret didn't really care for vegetables, so when she forced herself to eat salads, she typically loaded up a bowl full of bagged iceberg lettuce with croutons, bacon bits, and creamy dressing. She felt very virtuous for having added a "salad" to her dinner of pasta or potatoes or rice.

At each visit over several years — monthly at first, then every 3 months, then twice a year — I added another bit of information to educate Margaret on how to get more nutrients into her food and how to reduce the glycemic load of her meals and snacks. However, simply knowing what is healthy doesn't mean a person can change her lifelong habits and start *living* healthy. Margaret and I brainstormed at length to come up with some ideas that would really satisfy her dietary preferences and tastes. It certainly doesn't benefit a person to say, "Don't eat this and don't eat that," until everything they once enjoyed has been banished from the kitchen. It is far more effective to sit down with someone and really come to an understanding of what they enjoy eating, and then help them find a way to alter their favorites into something as healthy as possible. A person needs to both *like* what they are eating and also be able to *prepare* it reasonably.

It took several years, but that is just what we did. Margaret loved bread, pasta, crackers, cookies, and sweets. We found ways to keep her happy without a slice of toast for most of her breakfasts, so that on the weekends, she could enjoy a piece of toast when she had the time to prepare a vegetable stir-fry to enjoy it with. She liked the opuntia fruit juice smoothies we invented, mixed with some herbs and nutrients so that she could make it quickly and be off to work. Margaret found she was plenty satisfied eating cooked buckwheat, barley, or quinoa — all having more nutrients, fiber, and a lower glycemic index than pasta — served with a variety of different vegetable sauces for dinner. She grew to enjoy different sorts of more nourishing salads once we brainstormed and came up with ingredients she could really sink her teeth into, like raisins, chickpeas (garbanzo beans), steamed veggies chilled with a vinaigrette marinade, nuts, and so on.

Margaret lost 30 pounds (13.6 kg) the first year of our working together, 15 more pounds (6.8 kg) the second, and between 5 and 10 pounds (2.27 and 4.54 kg) each year for several years after that. In all fairness, in addition to Margaret's willingness to change her diet, much of her success could also be attributed to her impressive walking program. The diagnosis of diabetes had scared Margaret, and she was highly motivated to put some effort into her health. Her blood sugar returned to the normal range, as did her cholesterol. And best of all, her self-esteem and energy level soared. This case is an example of the insulin-resistant diabetes that often goes hand in hand with PCOS. It is also an example of a woman who had numerous symptoms but was never diagnosed with PCOS, an all-too-common occurrence.

Do I Have PCOS?

Many women have PCOS without knowing it. Polycystic ovarian syndrome, also known as polycystic ovary syndrome, is the most common hormone condition among women. Between 2% and 18% of all women in North America have PCOS, but these percentages may be understated because many women are not aware that they have PCOS, so the condition remains undiagnosed and under-reported. Few people know much about PCOS — not because this is a "woman's" condition, but because the many hormone reactions involved and the variations in presentation make it hard to understand. At first, just remembering the three words in the acronym can be challenging. Because PCOS symptoms are not obvious and are seldom discussed, it is sometimes referred to as a silent or invisible condition. There is no one cause of PCOS, and no one cure.

Nature or Nurture

PCOS is a condition of multiple hormonal imbalances, most of which are characterized by insulin resistance, elevated androgens, and dysfunctional thyroid hormones. While there are many causes of these hormonal imbalances, genetic predisposition combined with environmental factors may trigger the onset of PCOS. Research has shown that the genes involved with hormonal regulation can be over- or under-expressed — a phenomenon referred to as gene expression. Gene expression is affected not only by hereditary influences, but also by our diet, nutritional status, toxin load, and other environmental factors. Abnormal gene expression may lead to the complex hormone disruptions that characterize PCOS. These same abnormalities occur in diabetes and metabolic syndrome (related conditions that frequently occur in tandem with PCOS).

For some women, these genetic abnormalities are never expressed due to the balancing effects of a good diet and regular exercise. For other women, however, poor diet can trigger this genetic predisposition and initiate hormonal imbalances. Genes may be "turned on" or "turned off" by various lifestyle factors — and a pregnant woman's diet can even affect the genetic predisposition of her baby in utero.

PCOS facts

Serious Consequences

Approximately 50% of women with PCOS develop clinically evident diabetes or prediabetes, while 40% of women with PCOS develop high blood pressure. The risk of ovarian or endometrial cancers is three times as high in women with PCOS as in women without PCOS. Clearly, this condition needs to be taken seriously.

PCOS facts

Dietary Predisposition

PCOS occurs most frequently in developed countries and is less common in regions and cultures without access to or interest in refined sugar, processed grains, and junk foods. Although some components of the disorder appear to be hereditary, diet and lifestyle are instrumental in triggering genetic predisposition to PCOS.

The Female Reproductive System

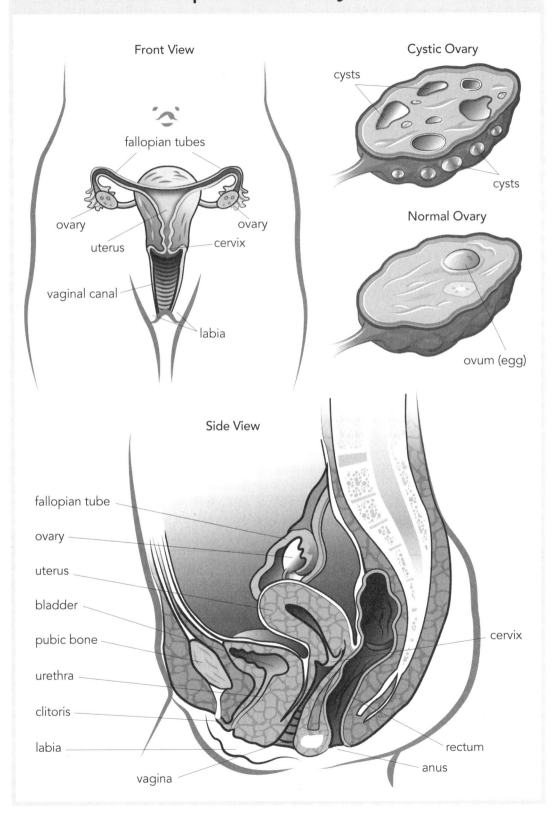

Front View

fallopian tubes

ovary

uterus

cervix

vaginal canal

labia

Cystic Ovary

cysts

cysts

Normal Ovary

ovum (egg)

Side View

fallopian tube

ovary

uterus

bladder

pubic bone

urethra

clitoris

labia

vagina

cervix

rectum

anus

How Can PCOS Be Defined?

The term "polycystic ovarian syndrome" may not just roll right off the tongue, but breaking down the four components of the acronym PCOS helps to define this condition. Refer to the illustration of the female reproductive system and the ultrasound images of normal and polycystic ovaries on page 12.

Poly

The prefix "poly-" means "many" or "more than one" — in this case, more than one ovarian cyst. The title is a slight misnomer, however, because not all women with PCOS have ovarian cysts.

Cystic

A cyst is a collection of fluid encased by a very thin wall of tissue, and the word "cystic" refers to a tissue or growth that contains cysts. Cysts can be functional or pathologic. Functional cysts form as a result of the normal function of the ovary as it goes through the various phases of the menstrual cycle. Functional cysts include follicular, corpus luteal, hemorrhagic, and endometrioid cysts. Pathologic cysts are the result of a disease process, such as PCOS, where there are often multiple pathologic cysts on the ovaries.

Follicular Cysts

Also called Graafian cysts, follicular cysts are the most common type of ovarian cysts. They may emerge and recede rather quickly over several months. These cysts are the result of an abnormal retention and growth of an ovarian follicle, the sac that releases an egg during the ovulatory phase of the menstrual cycle. The persistence of the ovarian follicle prevents the release of the egg and may lead to disturbances in the menstrual cycles, and, in some cases, pain. Any ovarian follicle that is larger than about $\frac{3}{4}$ inch (2 cm) in diameter is termed an ovarian cyst. In the case of PCOS and single-follicular cysts, the ripening egg is not released from the follicle, ovulation does not occur, and the cyst grows larger.

Corpus Luteal Cysts

The corpus luteum is the tiny group of cells left after a developed follicle containing an egg has risen to the surface of the ovary and released the egg into the fallopian tube. If pregnancy occurs, the corpus luteum does not scar over; instead, it persists and helps produce hormones to sustain a healthy pregnancy. In other cases, the corpus luteum develops into a cyst rather than scarring over.

Such cysts often cause no problems or symptoms and may eventually resolve on their own over several months. However, occasionally the cysts can grow to be quite large, filling with blood or fluid and reaching 4 inches (10 cm) in diameter. Large corpus luteum cysts may put such weight on the ovary that the ovary may twist inside the pelvic cavity, creating acute pain and becoming a surgical emergency.

Endometrioid Cysts

The endometrium is the inner lining of the uterus. It builds up each month and is shed with the menses. Endometriosis is a condition where the endometrial lining is displaced and begins growing in inappropriate places outside of the uterus. Endometrial cysts are cystic collections of endometrial tissue growing on the ovaries. They may be small and circular or in large patches. Endometrioid cysts often cause significant pelvic pain because menstrual blood may be released into the pelvic cavity, causing inflammation. Small endometrioid cysts are sometimes called "chocolate cysts" because the trapped blood has a chocolate brown color.

Ovarian

Women are born with two ovaries, located low in the pelvis on either side of the uterus and connected to the uterus via the fallopian tubes. They are the source of eggs, or ova, the woman's contribution to creating a new life. (Men possess testes, the source of sperm and the man's genetic contribution to a fertilized embryo.) The ovaries contain numerous follicles, spherical aggregations of cells containing eggs. Normally, just one egg develops, or ripens, inside a follicle each month, usually alternating between the left and right ovary. If one ovary is absent or dysfunctional, the other ovary will continue to release an egg. In PCOS, the ovaries often become enlarged due to the development and persistence of abnormal ova and follicles.

Syndrome

The term "syndrome" derives from the Greek and means "coming together." In medical parlance, a syndrome refers to a set of associated symptoms that occur together but whose cause has not yet been discovered. PCOS is called a syndrome rather than a disease because the diagnosis is based on a variety of symptoms and abnormalities that may or may not be present in all cases. This syndrome involves multiple hormonal disorders that can manifest as a collection of various symptoms that may be minor and vague — or may be significant and life-disrupting.

Endocrine System

PCOS is a condition involving the endocrine system. The word "endocrine" refers to the glands and organs that produce hormones. Hormones are typically released into the circulatory system to regulate specific bodily functions, such as metabolism and reproductive function, including ovulation. Hormones are transported to tissues where they bind with target receptors. Some hormones act locally near the gland that produces them, while others act remotely. Some hormones act on their own, while others are regulated by "releasing" hormones. The hypothalamus, a region in the brain, produces these releasing hormones, which act on the pituitary gland in another region in the brain. In turn, the pituitary releases numerous hormones that act more directly on target organs, such as the ovaries, but also the thyroid and adrenal glands, as well as other organs.

The Endocrine System

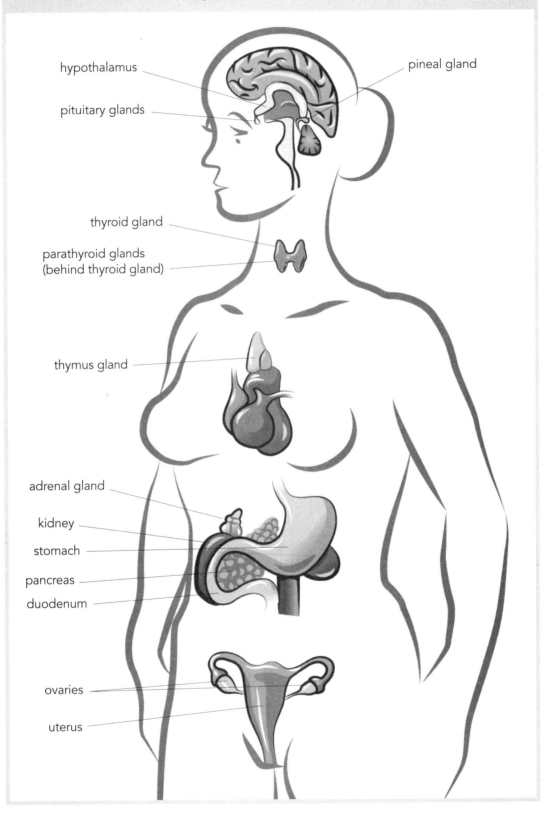

hypothalamus

pineal gland

pituitary glands

thyroid gland

parathyroid glands
(behind thyroid gland)

thymus gland

adrenal gland

kidney

stomach

pancreas

duodenum

ovaries

uterus

PCOS Problems in the Endocrine System

Gland/Organ	Hormone	Site of Action	Action	PCOS Problem
Anterior pituitary gland	Growth hormone (GH)	Most cells of the body	• Stimulates cell growth	
	Adrenocorticotropic hormone (ACTH)	Adrenal glands	• Stimulates adrenal cortex to release cortisol and aldosterone	
	Thyroid-stimulating hormone (TSH)	Thyroid gland	• Causes thyroid to secrete thyroid hormones	Irregular or disrupted feedback loop in PCOS
	Follicle-stimulating hormone (FSH)	Ovary, testes	• Promotes growth of follicles within the ovary (female) • Promotes formation of sperm (male)	Irregular or disrupted feedback loop in PCOS
	Luteinizing hormone (LH)	Ovary, testes	• Stimulates estrogen/progesterone release (female) • Stimulates testosterone release (male)	Irregular or disrupted feedback loop in PCOS
	Prolactin	Breast tissue	• Encourages breast development, milk production in pregnancy • Suppresses ovulation	Often elevated in PCOS, impairing ovulation and fertility
Posterior pituitary gland	Antidiuretic hormone (ADH)	Kidneys, blood vessels	• Causes kidneys to retain water • Increases blood pressure	
	Oxytocin	Uterus, breast tissue	• Induces contractions during labor, and milk expulsion	
Pineal gland	Melatonin	Brain, immune system	• Governs sleep/wake cycle	

PCOS Problems in the Endocrine System

Gland/Organ	Hormone	Site of Action	Action	PCOS Problem
Thyroid gland	Thyroxine (T4), triiodothyronine (T3)	Most cells of the body	• Increases metabolism, chemical reactions	Lowered in PCOS, or TSH receptors may be under-responsive
	Calcitonin	Bone cells	• Increases calcium deposition in bone, decreases levels in the blood	
Parathyroid glands	Parathormone	Gut, kidney, bone	• Increases calcium in the blood	
Adrenal glands (medulla)	Adrenaline and noradrenaline	Rapid response tissues	• Stimulates action and reaction (fight or flight mechanisms)	
Adrenal glands (cortex)	Dehydroepi-androsterone (DHEA), DHEA-S, and androstenedione Cortisol	Many cells and tissues	• Metabolic precursors to androgens and progesterone	Androgens elevated in PCOS
	Aldosterone	Kidneys, sweat glands	• Promotes sodium/water retention; increases potassium loss	
Pancreas	Insulin	Most cells of the body	• Promotes entry of sugar into cells • Involved in fat deposition	Increased insulin resistance in PCOS
	Glucagon	Liver, fat, muscle	• Increases glucose production and release into the blood	
Ovaries	Estrogens	Sex organs, uterus, bone	• Involved in sexual development, menstruation, uterine tissue buildup, bone metabolism	Disrupted in PCOS

PCOS Problems in the Endocrine System

Gland/Organ	Hormone	Site of Action	Action	PCOS Problem
Ovaries (continued)	Progesterone	Sex organs, uterus	• Involved in sexual development, menstruation, uterine secretion, pregnancy	Disrupted in PCOS
	Testosterone	Sex organs, adrenal glands	• Involved in sexual development (female), menstruation, uterine secretion, pregnancy	Disrupted in PCOS
Adipose tissue	Leptins, adipokines, adiponectin	Adipose tissue	• Regulate fat cells	Disrupted in PCOS
Hypothalamus (Although not considered an endocrine gland, the hypothalamus exerts control over the pituitary gland via neurohormones.)	Corticotropin-releasing hormone (CRH)	Anterior pituitary	• Stimulates release of ACTH	
	Growth hormone–releasing hormone	Anterior pituitary	• Stimulates release of GH	
	Gonadotropin-releasing hormone (GnRH)	Anterior pituitary	• Stimulates release of LH and FSH	Irregular or disrupted in PCOS
	Thyrotropin-releasing hormone (TRH)	Anterior pituitary	• Stimulates release of TSH	Irregular or disrupted in PCOS
	Prolactin inhibitory factor (dopamine)	Anterior pituitary	• Inhibits release of prolactin	Dopamine activity often low in PCOS

Source: Adapted with permission from Kendall-Reed P and Reed S. *The Complete Doctor's Stress Solution.* Toronto: Robert Rose Inc., 2004.

Feedback Loops

The endocrine system involves multiple signals and cross-talk among the various hormone-producing organs and the brain that increases (positive feedback) or decreases (negative feedback) hormone levels. Feedback loops enable the maintenance of endocrine equilibrium, or balance.

For example, in ovulation, an ovary secretes these sex hormones based on "feedback" information provided by the pituitary gland and the hypothalamus, located in the brain. When functioning properly, the hypothalamus releases gonadotropin-releasing hormone (GnRH), which tells the pituitary gland to release follicle-stimulating hormone (FSH) and luteinizing hormone (LH). FSH and LH travel in the bloodstream to the ovaries and stimulate them to make estrogen and progesterone. As estrogen or androgen levels in the bloodstream rise, they produce "negative feedback" to the

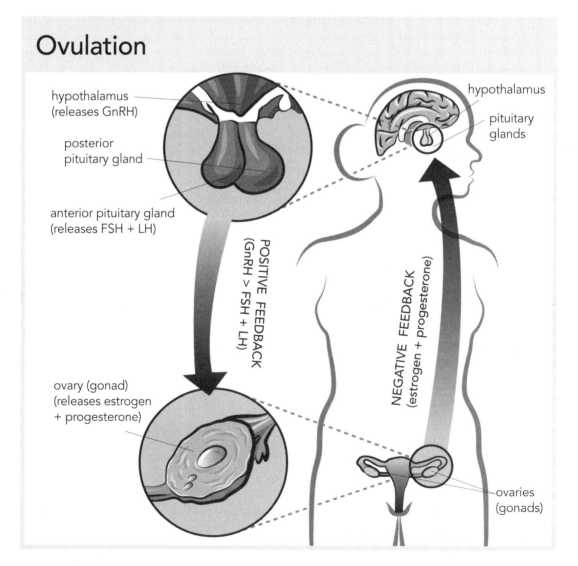

Ovulation

hypothalamus (releases GnRH)

posterior pituitary gland

anterior pituitary gland (releases FSH + LH)

hypothalamus

pituitary glands

POSITIVE FEEDBACK (GnRH > FSH + LH)

NEGATIVE FEEDBACK (estrogen + progesterone)

ovary (gonad) (releases estrogen + progesterone)

ovaries (gonads)

hypothalamus, causing it to halt the production and release of GnRH and adrenal-stimulating substances. This feedback loop between your ovaries and your brain is one way that hormones are controlled and balanced in your reproductive system.

The adrenal glands also make related sex hormones, specifically the androgens DHEA, DHEA-sulfate, and androstenedione, a precursor of testosterone and estrogen. Like the ovaries, hormone production in the adrenal glands is regulated via a feedback loop with the hypothalamus and pituitary gland in the brain. PCOS involves altered hormone levels, feedback loops, and tissue responses to hormones.

Elevated Androgens

Among the many hormones, androgens have the greatest impact on developing PCOS. Androgens include the steroid hormones dehydroepiandrosterone (DHEA), sometimes called the mother steroid; testosterone; and dihydrotestosterone and androstenedione.

Although men and women have androgens and estrogens, androgens are often referred to as the male hormones, and estrogens as the female hormones. Androgens are anabolic, meaning that they promote the storing of nutrients and the buildup of tissues. Androgens are a type of steroid, and, like all steroids, they are made out of cholesterol.

Men typically have higher androgen levels (particularly testosterone) than women, which contributes to more vigorous body hair and muscle mass in men. Women with high testosterone levels may develop facial hair and coarse and thick body hair. PCOS is characterized by having elevated androgens, contributing to infertility, menstrual disorders, and numerous complex hormonal imbalances.

Increased Insulin Resistance

PCOS studies have shown that high androgen levels are linked with insulin resistance — a phenomenon where cells do not respond to the hormone insulin as they should and are said to "resist" the influence of insulin. Research is revealing numerous abnormalities in the cellular response to insulin in women with PCOS.

Insulin is a hormone released by the pancreas into the bloodstream and travels via the circulatory system to the target organs and cells. Insulin is produced by the pancreas in special cells known as the beta cells in the islets of Langerhans. Insulin is released in response to the presence of glucose in the blood, with the goal of getting that glucose moved into cells. After you

PCOS facts

Testosterone Disturbances

Androgens, such as testosterone, are elevated in PCOS. Studies show that when animals are exposed to abnormally high levels of testosterone before puberty, they develop reproductive and metabolic disturbances consistent with those of PCOS in humans.

eat a meal, the ingested foods are broken down, and various fats, sugars, and amino acids from proteins are absorbed across the intestinal lining and into the blood stream. Insulin is crucial in helping to metabolize these compounds, moving them out of the blood and into the cells. As a result, insulin resistance can have serious metabolic consequences.

Gate Keepers

When insulin travels through the blood to target cells, it binds to special receptors on the outer surface of cell membranes and facilitates the entry of glucose into cells. Once inside various body cells, glucose may be used immediately as fuel or may be stored for future use. The liver and muscles in particular store large amounts of glucose by converting it to a starch known as glycogen.

When glucose is successfully moved into cells, the blood sugar drops and the pancreas stops producing insulin. If the cells do not take up the glucose successfully, as with insulin resistance, the blood sugar remains high and the pancreas continues to produce insulin. The more elevated blood insulin levels are, and the longer they remain elevated, the more resistant to insulin cells may become. This creates a vicious cycle.

Thyroid Irregularities

Thyroid disease is more common in women with PCOS than in other women, indicating that the complex endocrine imbalances involved with PCOS extend to the thyroid. It has long been known, for example, that many hypothyroid women suffer menstrual cycle irregularities, so commonly that this symptom is typically included in textbook symptom lists for hypothyroidism. Even more specifically, many hypothyroid women have been shown to have cysts on their ovaries when pelvic ultrasounds are performed, and sometimes these cysts will resolve when thyroid hormones are supplemented. Lack of regular monthly ovulation is another classic sign of hypothyroidism. Thyroid hormone therapy will sometimes restore monthly menses, normal ovulation, and fertility in hypothyroid women. All women with PCOS or suspected of having PCOS should have thyroid function tests run regularly, including a thyroid stimulating hormone (TSH) level.

PCOS facts

TSH Association with PCOS

Thyroid-stimulating hormone (TSH) is a hormone released from the pituitary where it travels in the blood and stimulates the thyroid gland. One study followed 103 women with PCOS and reported that hypothyroidism was closely correlated with the severity of insulin resistance and androgen elevation.

What Are the Symptoms of PCOS?

There is no one cause of PCOS and no one symptom that confirms diagnosis of this syndrome. Instead, it is a combination of symptoms that indicates the possible presence of PCOS. The syndrome is best characterized by elevated androgen levels. Menstrual irregularities and infertility in tandem with excessive hair growth, moderate to severe acne, and a variety of abnormal lab tests suggest the diagnosis of PCOS. In other cases, the menstrual cycles may be fairly normal, but obesity about the midsection, slight abnormalities in thyroid function, and abnormal insulin and glucose levels are indicative of PCOS.

Early or Late Menarche

Although many of the metabolic disorders that characterize PCOS are present long before puberty, the symptoms typically only manifest at the onset of puberty, when a young woman's menstrual cycles begin. Some women with PCOS may have an unusually early or unusually late menarche (onset of menses).

Irregular Menstrual Cycles

In PCOS, the menstrual cycles may be irregular or may be absent altogether, a condition referred to as amenorrhea. Some women may begin to menstruate normally and then develop irregular menses several years or even 10 years later as the hormone imbalances progress.

PCOS facts

Acne

Acne is a common symptom of PCOS. This inflammatory skin disorder involves interactions among hormones, hair, oil-secreting glands, and bacteria. Women with PCOS are susceptible, possibly due to excess levels of androgens.

Symptoms of PCOS

- Unusually early or unusually late menarche
- Irregular, infrequent, or absent menstrual cycles
- Increased facial and body hair
- Weight gain and central obesity
- Acne
- Infertility

NICHD Diagnostic Criteria

In 1990, the National Institute of Child Health and Human Disease (NICHD) established diagnostic criteria for PCOS:

1. Oligo-ovulation or anovulation manifested by oligomenorrhea and amenorrhea.

2. Hyperandrogenism (androgen excess) or hyperandrogenemia.

3. Polycystic ovaries (as defined by ultrasonography).

Weight Gain and Central Obesity

Due to a difficulty with basic metabolism, many women with PCOS struggle to maintain a healthy weight, even with rigorous exercise routines. Because there are different types of fat cells in the body and the fat cells in the trunk are most affected, women with PCOS often pack weight about their midsections and have relatively thin arms and legs.

Infertility

Many infertile women are ultimately found to have PCOS, and infertility evaluations may reveal multiple small cysts on both ovaries. Many women with irregular menstrual cycles are diagnosed as having PCOS, and having irregular menses interferes with fertility. When pregnancy does occur, women with PCOS suffer more complications in pregnancy and have an increased risk of miscarrying.

Q. I have started to grow coarse body hair. What causes this and what can I do to stop it?

A. Due to elevated amounts of androgens, such as testosterone, in the blood, many women with PCOS have hirsutism, or excessive facial and body hair. Testosterone promotes the growth of facial and body hair, and causes fine downy "peach fuzz" hair to become coarser and darker hair, like a man's whiskers. Many women with PCOS may sprout chin or upper lip hair and more vigorous body hair on the legs and even chest. Once a hair follicle begins to produce a coarser hair, there seems to be nothing that will reverse this, short of electrolysis. Many of the hormonal-balancing therapies discussed in this book, however, will help to decrease the conversion of peach fuzz hair follicles into coarse whiskers.

How Is PCOS Diagnosed?

There is no one test for PCOS, but several blood tests for abnormal hormone levels plus ultrasound examination of the ovaries may help confirm a diagnosis.

Elevated Androgen Levels

Patients with PCOS often have abnormally high levels of androgens, especially testosterone, in the blood.

Elevated Glucose, Insulin, and Cholesterol Levels

Blood tests may show higher than average levels of glucose, insulin, and cholesterol, all signs of possible insulin resistance.

Abnormal Thyroid

Blood tests may show abnormally low thyroid levels and/or the presence of unique antithyroid antibodies. Some women may display normal levels of thyroid hormones, but abnormally high TSH (thyroid-stimulating hormone) from the pituitary.

PCOS facts

Adiponectin

Adiponectin, a novel (recently discovered) hormone, is released from adipose (fat) tissue and helps direct fat cell metabolism. It is often involved in the development of obesity and hormone imbalance that are characteristic of most women with PCOS. Although it is not yet a diagnostic lab test, adiponectin levels are being noted as a sign of PCOS pathology.

Q. My mother is overweight and diabetic. She had a lot of trouble with miscarriages before she had me. Do you think she might have PCOS? And if she does, does it mean that I do too?

A. Hearing your mother's history, it is likely that she has some degree of the hormonal imbalances typical of PCOS. It is hard to say if you do too, but you are certainly predisposed to some of the same difficulties. By following the dietary, nutritional, and herbal advice in this book, you should be able to reduce your chances of developing diabetes and restore healthy hormonal balance.

Pituitary Hormones

Blood tests may show abnormal levels of regulating hormones from the pituitary, such as GnRH, TSH, FSH, LH, and prolactin.

Oversized Ovaries

As seen in pelvic ultrasound tests, the ovaries of women with PCOS are often larger than normal and may display multiple cysts. Using ultrasound imagery, multiple cysts can often be detected on the ovaries of girls as young as 10 to 18 years of age. Pelvic ultrasounds are being investigated as a possible screening tool in adolescents suspected of having PCOS.

Q. I fear I may have PCOS and have made an appointment with my doctor. What should I tell her?

A. You can help your doctor help you. Unfortunately, not all physicians recognize the more subtle presentations of PCOS. Even worse, it may not be understood that even the more subtle and vague presentations can cause the damage this syndrome can wreak if allowed to progress unrecognized. If you are struggling with infertility, irregular menses, weight gain, abnormal hair growth, and high blood sugar, ask your doctor about the possibility of PCOS so that appropriate tests can be run. Your physician will likely suggest blood work to check testosterone levels. Your doctor may also ask for a standard chemistry panel that looks at your fasting glucose, cholesterol, and blood fats. If your doctor doesn't suggest it, ask for a glucose tolerance test with insulin levels. This is more likely to catch minor difficulties with glucose regulation that simple spot checks may miss. A thyroid function panel that includes thyroid hormone levels, TSH, and thyroid antibodies is also appropriate.

Chapter 2

What Conditions Are Associated with PCOS?

CASE HISTORY

❧ *Rhonda*

When Rhonda first visited our clinic, she was 34 years old, a hardworking dairy farmer, happily married, with a great sense of humor. Rhonda and her husband had been married for 5 years and had been trying to have a child for the last 3. Rhonda came in to see me after receiving results from extensive lab work and examinations performed to evaluate fertility. She had been told that everything was "normal" and that she could consider a fertility specialist for possible pharmaceutical therapy or in vitro fertilization, albeit with the caveat that her insurance did not cover such things.

I looked at her blood work and noticed that a few important tests — prolactin and testosterone — had not yet been completed, and that a few findings in her "normal" lab tests were actually less than optimal. Rhonda's fasting glucose was 105 mg/dL (5.8 mmol/L), her lipids were all on the high end of the normal ranges, and her thyrotrophin (thyroid-stimulating hormone, or TSH) was just several points above the cut-off for the normal range. Additional lab testing of prolactin and testosterone found prolactin to be in the high normal range and testosterone to be slightly elevated.

Rhonda was having regular monthly menses. She had experienced moderate acne throughout her 20s and still suffered occasional pimples that would emerge painfully and take many weeks to fully resolve. Despite a very high activity level on her farm, she packed a bit of weight about her abdomen. She was otherwise quite healthy, rarely ill, and had good energy. She slept well and had no other significant health complaints. She ate a fairly healthy diet, although it could be improved upon by adding more fresh vegetables and by eliminating the evening cookies and ice cream and replacing them with something healthier, such as fresh fruit.

We discussed a simple game plan of using herbs and nutrients for a full year and then taking note of any change before continuing on with expensive lab work and consultations with specialists. We began an herbal tincture of *Vitex agnus-castus*, *Angelica sinensis*, *Serenoa repens*, and *Polygonum multiflorum*, plus a multi-B vitamin, vitamin D, and cod liver oil. We also put together an herbal tea for her to drink whenever possible, hot or cold. We sent her home with opuntia juice to add to her tea, to prepare a spritzer with sparkling mineral water, or to put in a morning fruit smoothie, as desired.

Rhonda called me after just 8 weeks. Her menses was 1 week late. Because many women with PCOS have irregular menses, I was less sure, but a visit to my office the next day yielded a positive pregnancy test.

Sadly, Rhonda miscarried a month later. It appeared that the nutritional and herbal protocol was improving fertility, but perhaps we should wait until a more solid hormonal balance had been achieved before attempting pregnancy again, perhaps in 6 months. Rhonda reluctantly saw the logic of this and 5 months later called again to say that her menses was overdue. A pregnancy test confirmed the pregnancy, and this time Rhonda carried the baby to full term. She delivered a healthy boy in the spring — on the same schedule as her cows.

Preventive Measures

The metabolic and hormonal imbalances associated with PCOS may also lead to diabetes, heart disease, and reproductive cancers. Women with PCOS are at risk of becoming diabetic; problems with insulin response and blood sugar regulation are associated with both conditions. An inability to metabolize sugar and fats can also lead to high cholesterol, high blood pressure, and ultimately heart disease. Obesity is also associated with altered blood sugar and fats seen in many women with PCOS and insulin resistance. For some women, sluggish thyroid function may contribute to PCOS and obesity, compounding the problem of insulin resistance. The hormonal and metabolic imbalances that are typical of PCOS also put women at risk for reproductive cancers, such as breast and ovarian cancer.

Due to these numerous and serious associated conditions, diagnosing hormonal and metabolic imbalances as early as possible is an important preventive measure. Making some healthy lifestyle changes can help prevent PCOS from progressing to heart disease, diabetes, and cancer.

Conditions Associated with PCOS

- Abnormal menstruation
- Infertility
- Diabetes mellitus type 2
- Metabolic syndrome
- Chronic obesity
- Heart disease
- Thyroid disease
- Ovarian cancer
- Endometrial cancer

PCOS Risk Factors

PCOS is a risk factor for many serious diseases and disorders. Effectively managing PCOS lowers the possible incidence of these challenges to your good health.

Genetic Expression / Environmental Impact
▼
Disrupted or Irregular Pituitary
Hormone Release and Feedback
▼
Elevated Androgens / Increased
Insulin Resistance / Thyroid Imbalance
▼
PCOS
▼
Abnormal Menstruation / Infertility / Diabetes /
Metabolic Syndrome / Chronic Obesity /
Heart Disease / Thyroid Disease / Hormonal Cancer

Abnormal Menstruation

The hormone irregularities that characterize PCOS contribute to all forms of abnormal menstruation and to an irregular menstrual cycle. Restoring regular menses is one step in managing PCOS.

Menarche

"Menarche" refers to the first time a woman menstruates. Both abnormally early and abnormally late menarche may result from the hormonal imbalances associated with PCOS. The onset of menses involves coordinated changes in hypothalamic, pituitary, and reproductive hormones, and may be interfered with due to abnormally high androgen or prolactin levels, or simply subtle imbalances in the whole big picture.

Amenorrhea

"Amenorrhea" is a term meaning the abnormal suppression, or absence, of menses, and many women with PCOS experience this cessation due to elevated testosterone and especially prolactin levels.

Dysmenorrhea

"Dysmenorrhea" refers to difficult or painful menses. Dysmenorrhea involves menstrual cramping and pain and can be caused by PCOS. Elevated levels of prostaglandins and other inflammatory compounds contribute to dysmenorrhea.

Menorrhagia

Sometimes women experience excessive bleeding, or menorrhagia, during menstruation. This may be caused by excessive buildup of the uterine lining, the presence of uterine fibroids and polyps, or problems with the tone of the uterine muscle. Excessive levels of estrogen and lack of opposing progesterone can contribute to menorrhagia.

Menopause

Menopause is the cessation of regular monthly menses and usually occurs around the age of 50. The menopausal transition may involve irregular menstrual cycles, hot flashes, insomnia,

---

PCOS facts

PMS and PCOS

In premenstrual syndrome (PMS), a woman experiences various hormonally induced symptoms prior to her menstrual period, such as intestinal bloating, breast tenderness, headache, fluid retention, mood swings, and emotional irritability. All such symptoms typically resolve with the onset of the menses. As with PCOS, excessive levels of estrogen or the lack of opposing progesterone may contribute to PMS. Nutritional deficiencies and poor health of the liver and digestive system may also contribute to PMS.

---

and emotional disturbances. Menopause involves a decline in all reproductive hormones, including estrogen, progesterone and the androgens. The analogous decline of reproductive hormones in men is referred to as andropause.

Infertility

Along with uterine fibroids, endometriosis, and blocked fallopian tubes, PCOS is among the leading causes of female infertility.

Hormone imbalances

Women with PCOS may have difficulty becoming pregnant due to complex hormonal imbalances that interfere with the maturation of eggs in the ovarian follicles. Any one hormonal abnormality can interfere with fertility, and with PCOS, there are usually multiple imbalances of elevated androgens, insulin, and prolactin. The ovaries may be incapable of maturing and releasing an egg, or — when ovulation and fertilization do occur — the hormonal imbalances may interfere with maintaining the pregnancy. Miscarriages are common.

Thyroid Dysfunction in PCOS

There is a strong correlation between autoimmune hypothyroid disorders and infertility. Thyroid hormones have an impact on all reproductive organs and they affect reproductive hormones in numerous direct and indirect ways. Hypothyroidism is also associated with miscarriages and infertility. Supporting healthy thyroid function may also improve fertility and support positive pregnancy outcomes.

Ovarian Circulation

Women with high androgen levels and cysts on the ovaries may also have poor circulation in the endometrium, the blood-rich lining of the uterus. This impairment of circulation may be another factor contributing to infertility and early miscarriages. Although there is little modern research on the subject, *Angelica sinensis* has been used for centuries in traditional Chinese medicine to improve circulation in the pelvis, including the uterus and ovaries. *Polygonum multiflorum* and *Leonurus sibiricus* are other medicinal herbs believed to improve fertility and circulation in the pelvis. Herbalists and naturopathic physicians may prescribe fertility-enhancing herbal formulas that include these circulatory agents for women with PCOS.

PCOS facts

Clinical Definition of Infertility

Infertility is defined as an inability to conceive despite one full year of unprotected intercourse. The most common cause of infertility in men is having a low sperm count and/or abnormal sperm morphology. In women, ovarian causes, such as PCOS, may be to blame in around 25% of all infertility cases, and uterine disorders, such as uterine fibroids, endometriosis, and blocked fallopian tubes, in another 25%. Blocked fallopian tubes caused by a history of pelvic infections and sexually transmitted diseases may also occur. Approximately 10% of infertility cases may have no identifiable cause, and subtle hormonal imbalances may play a role in such cases.

Pregnancy Complications

Women with PCOS can experience other complications with full-term pregnancies, such as a greater risk of pregnancy-related high blood pressure and giving birth to an infant with jaundice. The general maternal fatality rate is higher in women with PCOS than in other women postpartum. The occurrence of gestational diabetes, premature labor, and stillbirth is higher in women with PCOS. Women with PCOS may also deliver larger infants or require C-sections more often than women without PCOS.

Blood Fat (Lipid) Processing

The abnormal processing of blood fats and cholesterol may also contribute to infertility. Obese women with PCOS have been found to have higher levels of oxidized low-density lipoprotein (LDL) cholesterol in their ovarian follicles than lean women and women without PCOS. This is believed to contribute to infertility and poor embryo health when pregnancy does occur.

Fertility Therapies

The most common therapies for infertility involve the use of hormonal medications that support ovulation and help prevent miscarriage. In vitro fertilization, where a woman's ova are fertilized outside the body with her husband's or a donor's sperm and then implanted in the hormone-prepped uterus, is one of the more extreme and expensive approaches. In vitro fertilization has a high failure rate but is sometimes successful in helping an infertile couple to have a child genetically their own when simpler measures have failed.

Other, less invasive natural therapies include dietary modification, nutritional and herbal supplementation, and exercise. When women optimize their diets, take hormone-balancing herbs and nutrients, and adopt a regular exercise routine over a "prenatal year," the results may be even better, although studies proving this are lacking.

Clomiphene (Clomid) for Fertility

This fertility drug stimulates the ovaries to ovulate and release an egg into the fallopian tubes. Many women with PCOS, however, do not respond as expected to clomiphene. Half of women with PCOS will ovulate with clomiphene drug therapy, but the other half will not and are said to be clomiphene resistant. (The presence of antithyroid peroxidase antibodies in the blood of women with PCOS may be a predictor of poor treatment response to clomiphene.) Many women who do not respond to clomiphene are found to have autoimmune hypothyroidism.

The simultaneous use of metformin, an antidiabetic drug, with clomiphene in women with PCOS has shown some promise in improving the success rate of in vitro fertilization as well as in reducing the miscarriage rate. Clomiphene should only be used for 6 months because it may actually impair fertility with long-term use and may increase the risk of ovarian cancer when used for 12 or more consecutive menstrual cycles. Clomiphene may also cause digestive upset, dizziness, headache, and visual disturbances. Because of these possible side affects and because the research on potential benefits is not complete, some authorities question its use.

Myo-inositol and *D-chiro-inositol*

Myo-inositol and *D-chiro-inositol* are inositol compounds that play a role in fertility and are involved in the maturation of immature follicles in the ovaries, promoting their growth into mature eggs to be released in monthly ovulation.

Myo-inositol levels have been found to be abnormally low in the ovarian follicles of women with PCOS. Supplementation with *Myo-inositol* or *D-chiro-inositol* may improve fertility in women with PCOS, as might the consumption of more foods with *D-chiro-inositol*, such as legumes. Legumes also support healthy levels of blood sugar and fat.

PCOS facts

Pituitary and Hypothalamic Hormones

When clomiphene fails, the use of pituitary and hypothalamic hormones may be successful, but this course of therapy is sometimes long and expensive, and multiple pregnancies (twins, triplets, quadruplets) may result. Women who do not respond to clomiphene are commonly found to have autoimmune hypothyroidism, and the presence of antithyroid peroxidase antibodies in the blood of women with PCOS may be a predictor of poor treatment response to clomiphene. Fertility specialists may use this information to help choose who will and who will not benefit from clomiphene medication.

One clinical study administered *myo-inositol* and vitamin B complex to women with PCOS and reported that elevated testosterone levels declined and ovulation was greatly improved. For patients undergoing in vitro fertilization, the health of collected eggs was also reported to improve following *myo-inositol* supplementation. Because inositol compounds have no known toxicity or significant side effect, they may be placed on the list of safe supplements for a woman with PCOS.

Prenatal Preparation

If you have PCOS and are planning a pregnancy, take several months, even a year, to prepare yourself. Improve your fertility and decrease the chance of miscarriage by improving your diet and by taking key supplements. If you have PCOS, your prenatal year diet and supplements might include the following:

- High-protein foods
- Limited refined carbohydrate foods
- Folic acid
- B vitamins
- Vitamin D
- Chromium
- Magnesium
- N-acetylcysteine
- *Myo-inositol* or *D-chiro-inositol*
- Maca powder in smoothies
- Brewer's yeast in food or smoothies
- Prickly pear juice

Hormonal Treatment Options

There are several hormones that can be injected to improve fertility. Again, the challenge is to restore hormonal balance and insure that this approach does not backfire by further unbalancing the endocrine system.

Human Chorionic Gonadotropin (HCG)

HCG is marketed under the brand names of Profasi and Pregnyl. HCG is given by injection. It is important to administer the injection during a time that takes other hormonal rhythms in the body into consideration. HCG stimulates the ovaries to release the most mature egg from the most developed follicle. Too much HCG, however, can over-stimulate the ovaries and lead to cyst formation rather than ovulation.

Herbal Tea for Infertility in PCOS

Ingredients (dried leaves and flowers)

- Alfalfa leaves (*Medicago sativa*)
- Raspberry leaves (*Rubus idaeus*)
- Stevia leaf (*Stevia rebaudiana*)
- Hibiscus flowers (*Hibiscus sabdariffa*)

1. Combine equal parts of the herbs (available in herb shops). Because you will be drinking it daily over a long term, you will need at least 4 or more ounces (120 g) of each herb to last any length of time.

2. Into a teapot or other vessel with a lid, add 1 rounded tablespoon (15 mL) of mixture per cup (250 mL) of boiling water and let herbs steep, covered, for 10 minutes. Strain and drink.

Note: You may drink as much as you like, but aim for at least 3 cups (750 mL) per day for optimal medicinal effects.

Herbal Tincture for Infertility in PCOS

Ingredients (tinctures are concentrated extracts of plants in a solution of alcohol)

- *Angelica sinensis* tincture
- *Polygonum multiflorum* tincture
- *Leonurus cardiaca* tincture
- *Vitex agnus-castus* tincture
- *Serenoa repens* tincture

1. Combine equal parts of the liquid tinctures and take 1 teaspoon (5 mL) three times daily.

Note: Herbalists and physicians can customize a formula to suit specific patients. Consult a physician regarding the continued use of these herbs should pregnancy occur.

Follicle-Stimulating Hormone (FSH) Injections

FSH is normally released from the pituitary gland in a precisely controlled rhythm. In a healthy menstrual cycle, the ebb and flow of FSH has a pattern that complements the ebb and flow of luteinizing hormone (LH). Some women with PCOS have excessive LH, and supplementing FSH in precisely timed injections may improve ovulation and fertility.

Gonadotropin-Releasing Hormone (GnRH)

GnRH is produced in the hypothalamus gland and acts on the pituitary gland to release reproductive hormones, which, in turn, act on the reproductive organs. If clomiphene has failed, there are natural and synthetic GnRH medications that may be tried. The timing and dosing of these medications is tricky, the therapy may be expensive, and there may be many side affects due to the numerous hormonal effects of GnRH.

Diabetes

Insulin resistance is a component of hormonal imbalances in half of women with PCOS. Insulin resistance is both a precursor to and a sub-set of diabetes, and it is often a subtle part of PCOS metabolic difficulties. Therapies that improve insulin response will not only help women with PCOS lose weight and restore fertility and reproductive function, they can also reduce the risk of heart disease and the risk of progressing to the full diabetic state.

Metabolizing Glucose

Glucose is one of the main sugars found in the body. We may eat sugar in the form of sucrose (cane sugar), lactose (milk sugar), and many other sugars or saccharides, but ultimately the body transforms these sugars into glucose. Even carbohydrates that do not taste obviously sweet, such as grains, will all ultimately be broken down into glucose. Glucose is often elevated in women with PCOS.

Insulin Assistance and Resistance

Glucose requires the assistance of insulin to enter cells. In some cases of PCOS, the cells do not respond well to insulin. In fact, insulin levels may be abnormally high in women with PCOS. If the cells do not respond to insulin, glucose remains in the bloodstream, where it contributes to pathological changes in the blood vessels and tissues.

Normally, insulin prompts cells to take in glucose and metabolize it to do whatever that cell does. Glucose is one of the most basic energy sources for cells: liver cells can store it as glycogen, muscle cells may "burn" or use it to contract and work, and the brain will metabolize it to think. When cells don't respond to insulin, basic metabolism in every tissue suffers. Insulin resistance causes more glucose to remain in the blood due to the inability to enter cells.

"Insulin resistance" is a medical term referring to the phenomenon where the cells "resist" the influence of insulin. Insulin resistance can lead to diabetes. Diabetes mellitus is a condition involving an abnormal elevation of glucose in the bloodstream.

Pancreas and Insulin Action

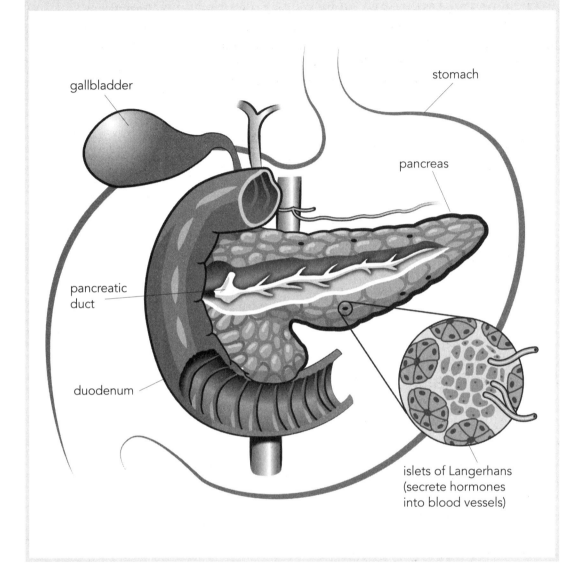

gallbladder

stomach

pancreas

pancreatic duct

duodenum

islets of Langerhans (secrete hormones into blood vessels)

Diabetes Incidence and Prevalence

Diabetes mellitus affects approximately 250 million people worldwide. The World Health Organization predicts that close to 400 million people will be living with diabetes by the year 2025. Although all regions of the world are affected, India, China, and the United States rank first, second, and third, respectively, which is due in part to the high population of these countries.

Defining Diabetes

Diabetes mellitus is commonly referred to as diabetes or sugar diabetes. The word "mellitus" means "sweet." Physicians used to taste the urine of people suspected of being diabetic because it would taste sweet. In diabetes mellitus, some of the unabsorbed glucose in the bloodstream is pulled out of the blood by the kidneys and ends up in the urine, a condition referred to as glucosuria, or sugar in the urine.

Type 1 and Type 2 Diabetes

There are two chief types of diabetes mellitus. In type 1 diabetes, the pancreas makes too little insulin and this lack of insulin impairs the uptake of glucose by the cells. This type of diabetes is associated with autoimmune, viral, drug, or other damage to the pancreatic beta cells that produce insulin. Type 1 diabetes is the less common form of diabetes, accounting for approximately 10% of all diabetes mellitus cases. Because insulin levels are low, this type of diabetic person almost always requires insulin supplementation. Type 1 diabetes is not caused by a faulty diet, although dietary measures are extremely important therapeutic considerations that can prolong life and prevent organ and tissue damage over time.

Diabetes Complications

The World Health Organization has reported the following statistics showing the impact of diabetes on other health conditions and diseases:

- Increased risk of heart disease and stroke (50% of people with diabetes will die of cardiovascular disease)
- Increased risk of foot ulcers and limb amputations
- Increased risk of blindness (2% of all people with diabetes will go blind and 10% will suffer significant visual impairment)
- Increased risk of kidney failure (10% to 20% of people with diabetes will die of kidney failure)
- Increased risk of nerve damage (about 50% of all people with diabetes will suffer numbness, tingling, and other symptoms of nerve damage)
- Increased risk of a shortened lifespan (overall risk of death at an early age is double for the diabetic population compared to the non-diabetic population)

Type 2 diabetes is usually not due to a lack of insulin production in the pancreas; rather, this condition occurs because of insulin resistance. This more common type of diabetes comprises approximately 90% of all diabetes mellitus cases. Because insulin levels are usually adequate, or often elevated, the majority of people with type 2 diabetes do not need insulin injections.

Type 2 diabetes often begins with minor insulin resistance, which progresses to the point where cells are so resistant to insulin that the blood sugar is abnormally elevated and falls within the diabetic range. Because the effort to produce so much insulin can stress the pancreas and cells, and because the high levels of glucose and lipids may cause pathologic changes, insulin resistance can lead to pancreatic and beta cell changes over time.

Type 1 and Type 2 Diabetes

Type 1 Diabetes: Insufficient insulin production, resulting in abnormally high blood sugar

Type 2 Diabetes: Sufficient insulin production, but inadequate cellular response to insulin, resulting in abnormally high blood sugar

Long-Term Complications of Diabetes

The presence of abnormally high sugar and fat in the bloodstream can do substantial damage to cells, tissues, and organs over time. Women with PCOS may also have abnormally high levels of blood fats and sugars due to insulin resistance and other metabolic imbalances.

Infections

Because the high sugar level in the blood creates an hospitable environment for bacteria, viruses, and fungi, many people with diabetes are plagued by frequent skin and bladder infections. Frequent colds and flu, sore throats, and vague malaise may occur as well, because most microbes thrive in a high-sugar environment. Controlling the elevated blood sugar as well as providing immune and nutritional support may help people with diabetes and women with PCOS with this these infections. Topical antifungal agents, such as tea tree oil, can be useful for chronic skin fungus, and boric acid vaginal suppositories or herbal douches may help women with chronic yeast vaginitis, although these treatments will not correct the underlying high blood sugar causing the problem.

Retinopathy

Some people with diabetes experience damage to the retina of the eyes; when untreated, this can lead to blindness. Vascular tonics are appropriate for all people with diabetes, to help protect the blood vessels from damage. *Allium sativum*, *Vaccinium myrtillis*, and *Ginkgo biloba* are agents that may help protect the tiny blood vessels of the eyes from being damaged by high blood fats and sugars.

Nephropathy

Damage to the tiny blood vessels in the kidney can lead to the destruction of individual glomeruli (tiny capillaries that help clean the blood), which slowly impairs the ability of the kidneys to filter the blood. Ultimately, destruction of the renal tissue can progress to kidney failure, which forces patients to undergo periodic dialysis to filter their blood using machines. In fact, the majority of patients requiring dialysis are diabetic. *Pueraria mirifica* and *Silybum marianum* are two herbs that may help protect the kidney cells and tiny blood vessels of the glomeruli from being damaged.

PCOS facts

Glucose Bombardment

Many women with PCOS show some degree of insulin resistance and are at risk of developing type 2 diabetes. Type 2 diabetes is very much associated with diet and a high intake of sugar (or of simple carbohydrates that quickly digest into sugar), which contributes to the progression of insulin resistance. The more a cell is bombarded with glucose (and, in turn, the higher the insulin levels), the more insulin resistant the cell may become.

Q. I have PCOS and I am diabetic. Sometimes I feel a tingling in my toes and fingers. Should I be concerned?

A. Yes, this could be an early sign of neuropathy, which occurs in some cases due to poor circulation to the limbs. Diabetes can destroy our tiniest blood vessels, the terminal capillary beds. As capillaries are destroyed, the delivery of oxygen to the fingers, toes, lips, and nose is impaired, and nerve endings become inflamed and die painfully due to the lack of circulation. Herbal agents, such as *Angelica sinensis* and *Gingko biloba*, may help deliver more oxygen to our limbs and microcirculatory vessels, helping to prevent and treat neuropathy.

Cutaneous Ulceration

Some people with diabetes develop chronic non-healing ulcers in the lower limbs. *Calendula officinalis* and *Gingko biloba* are among the herbal supplements that can improve skin health and promote the healing of wounds in people with diabetes. Calendula may support microcirculation in the skin itself, while gingko may help more blood, and thereby oxygen, reach the limbs.

Cardio and Peripheral Vascular Damage

Elevated glucose and lipids in the blood lead to inflammatory and oxidative processes that damage the blood vessels and heart tissue. As the blood vessels lose their elasticity, blood pressure may increase, and the risk of myocardial infarction (heart attack), stroke, and peripheral vascular diseases increase greatly. *Gingko biloba* and *Crataegus oxyacantha* may improve the delivery of oxygen to the heart and blood vessels.

Diagnosing Diabetes

There are several methods for diagnosing type 1 and type 2 diabetes.

Fasting Blood Sugar Levels

One way that diabetes mellitus can be diagnosed is by checking for elevated blood sugar levels after fasting, and checking on multiple occasions. Normal fasting blood glucose is between 70 and 90 mg/dL (3.9 and 5.0 mmol/L). Those whose fasting blood sugar is over 100 are said to have "impaired" glucose control, and those with a fasting glucose level of over 125 mg/dL (7.0 mmol/L) are diagnosed as diabetic. Some physicians may also check glucose levels 2 hours after eating, to assess the stability of the blood sugar level following the challenge of a meal.

The careful physician will know that any blood sugar above 100 in a fasting state is slightly elevated and may want to investigate further, especially if there are symptoms of PCOS in a woman. Doing so could help prevent the progression of impaired glucose tolerance to diabetes.

HbA1c

Another lab assessment of blood glucose regulation is a test known as HbA1c, also referred to as glycosylated hemoglobin. It is an indirect measure of long-term blood glucose control. An HbA1c test is often used to assess the general blood sugar control or to gauge results of various diabetes therapies.

Glucose Tolerance Tests

The glucose tolerance test (GTT), also called the oral glucose tolerance test (OGTT), is a more sensitive test in diagnosing poor blood sugar control and diabetes than random fasting blood glucose testing. With glucose tolerance testing, a higher percentage of people are identified as diabetic or as having impaired glucose control than by spot-checking fasting glucose levels alone. The reason for this is because the GTT doses a person with a high sugar load and draws blood multiple times over several hours to follow the rise and fall of the blood sugar level, whereas fasting glucose testing only takes one sample. Sometimes people who eat a healthy diet and have never received an abnormal blood sugar reading will show a transient abnormality with a GTT.

PCOS facts

Get Tested

People with PCOS who have abnormally elevated fasting glucose levels above 100 mg/dL (5.6 mmol/L), even though not in the diabetic range, should undergo a follow-up glucose tolerance test. This test may help identify poor blood sugar control and help diagnose diabetes in a way that checking fasting blood sugar levels failed to detect. If you have a family history of diabetes, if you smoke, and if you have simultaneous high blood pressure and cholesterol, take action because impaired glucose tolerance is also a risk factor for developing and dying from cardiovascular disease.

Q. How is a GTT performed?

A. Most doctors will ask patients to consume a sugar drink, typically 2½ ounces (75 g) of glucose dissolved into 1 cup (250 mL) water. (Some physicians may prefer asking a patient to eat a more typical but large and heavy meal and observing what happens to the blood sugar over the next several hours.) Healthy blood glucose control will manifest as a gradual and moderate rise in glucose, which begins to fall quickly as the resulting rise in insulin moves the absorbed glucose into cells. Within several hours of drinking the glucose beverage, the glucose should settle out to normal levels once again.

When there is poor glucose tolerance, the glucose may spike up quickly into the diabetic or near-diabetic range, and if insulin is not capable of moving the glucose into cells, the blood sugar may remain high 2 hours after the glucose was ingested.

Those who have a 2-hour glucose reading above 200 mg/dL (11.1 mmol/L) may be diagnosed as diabetic. Those with a 2-hour glucose level of 140 to 199 mg/dL (7.8 to 11.0 mmol/L) are said to have impaired glucose tolerance and may go on to become diabetic over time. A glucose tolerance test in the impaired range is also associated with an increased risk of cardiovascular disease, according to the World Health Organization. Some authorities argue that a cutoff of 180 mg/dL (10.0 mmol/L) for a 2-hour glucose tolerance test is a better criterion of diagnosing the diabetic state, because this level seems to bear the same cardiovascular and disease risks as those with 2-hour glucose readings of over 200 mg/dL.

Quantitative Insulin Sensitivity Check Index

The quantitative insulin sensitivity check index (QUICKI) is a laboratory measurement of insulin sensitivity. It's basically a glucose tolerance test partnered with an insulin check. This lab test involves measuring both the glucose and insulin levels in the blood, both fasting and 2 hours after consuming the glucose drink, to assess how much insulin is released and how effective the released insulin is in moving the glucose into the cells. Type 1 diabetics will show no insulin rise following the glucose challenge because their pancreas in unable to produce enough of the hormone. Type 2 diabetics usually show either a normal or an excessively high rise in insulin along with an abnormally high glucose level. Many women with PCOS display abnormally high QUICKI measurements.

Treatments for Diabetes

Although dietary therapy, nutrient supplements, and medicinal herbs are the best long-term strategies for managing diabetes, there are several effective drug therapies.

Biguanide Medications

Biguanide drugs have been used for type 2 diabetes for several decades, and research is starting to show that they can be an effective treatment option for women with PCOS. Metformin (Glucophage) is a biguanide that has been shown to promote ovulation, reduce insulin resistance, and improve the efficacy of fertility drugs. When used during pregnancy, metformin may reduce the tendency to miscarry. Metformin is not known to cause birth defects.

PCOS facts

Metformin and PCOS

One study involving a group of 30 women with both insulin resistance and PCOS investigated the effects of metformin therapy. The study participants were divided into two groups and both received diet and exercise advice. Half of the participants received 1,500 milligrams of metformin per day, and the other received half a placebo. Progress was tracked for both groups over 4 months, and participants were evaluated for any effects on menstrual cycles, hirsutism (excessive hair growth or distribution), and waist-to-hip ratios. Serum hormones, glucose, insulin, and blood fats were also evaluated. Statistically significant improvements in insulin and testosterone levels were seen only in the group that received the metformin, and these participants also experienced a notable reduction in waist-to-hip ratios and an improvement in the regularity of menstrual cycles. Other hormones were not impacted and hirsutism did not develop.

Mechanism of Action

Metformin may enhance the reception of insulin into the cells via a mechanism that involves adenosine monophosphate (AMP). Cyclic AMP-activated enzymes are also known as protein kinases, and they modify proteins by chemically adding phosphate groups to them. Cyclic AMP is found just inside the cell membrane and is sometimes called the "second messenger" because it is an intracellular molecule that helps send the message to protein kinase enzymes that insulin has docked and has bound insulin receptors on the outer cell surface. The protein kinase enzymes play their own role in perpetuating the domino cascade of biochemical responses inward to the nucleus of the cell. Nutrients, such as *D-chiro-inositol* and *pinitol*, may work in similar ways.

Metformin is not without its own risks. On rare occasions, metformin may induce damage to the kidneys and promote acute metabolic distress necessitating hospitalization. Consult a physician to see if you are a candidate that might benefit from metformin.

Inositol

Various forms of inositol may play a role in helping cells receive insulin and transmit the signal to the interior of the cell, where the nucleus and other organelles may respond in turn. Insulin resistance may be caused by a faulty signaling pathway that involves inositol-containing phosphoglycan molecules associated with cell membranes. *D-chiro-inositol* and the related substance *pinitol* occur naturally in some foods, including legumes and buckwheat. *D-chiro-inositol* may also be taken as a supplement.

Metabolic Syndrome

Metabolic syndrome is a pronounced type of insulin resistance, where insulin, blood glucose, and lipid levels are significantly elevated. As the condition progresses, blood pressure becomes elevated as well. Metabolic syndrome is associated with a significantly increased risk of heart disease and damage to the heart organ.

Metabolic syndrome is also referred to as metabolic cardiovascular syndrome, metabolic syndrome of obesity, and insulin resistance syndrome. The International Diabetes Federation has called the combination of symptoms — hypertension, high blood sugar, high cholesterol, and obesity — the Deadly Quartet. Like diabetes, it appears that genetic predispositions do exist in metabolic syndrome but that diet and lifestyle are equally important triggers for the condition.

The insulin resistance in metabolic syndrome may emerge as early as pre-puberty. The buildup of fats in the arteries that leads to coronary heart disease and stroke may begin at this time as well. People who suffer heart attacks at a very young age may have had metabolic syndrome for most of their lives. Metabolic syndrome may also be associated with a predisposition to certain cancers, Alzheimer's disease, and other forms of dementia.

The Deadly Quartet

1. High blood pressure
2. High blood sugar
3. High cholesterol
4. Obesity

Signs and Symptoms of Metabolic Syndrome

- Early and excessive weight gain during childhood
- Persistent adult obesity
- High blood pressure, high cholesterol, and high blood sugar
- Premature puberty
- Allergies
- Breast enlargement in men
- Fat accumulation in the liver
- Early and severe development of atherosclerosis (inflammatory damage and tissue changes in the arteries)
- Blood-clotting disorders
- Chronic inflammatory disorders, such as gout or skin rashes (chronic inflammation itself is also associated with an increased risk of cancer and dementia)

PCOS facts

The Journal of the American Medical Association has reported that 22% to 24% of the United States general population could be diagnosed with metabolic syndrome, with approximately 7% of people in their 20s and more than 40% of people in their 60s being affected. Men and women are equally affected, except in African American and Mexican American populations, where women are more affected.

Conditions Associated with Metabolic Syndrome

- Ovarian cysts
- PCOS
- Obesity
- Chronic inflammatory disorder
- Atherosclerosis
- Fatty liver
- Blood clots
- Gout
- Dermatitis
- Dementia and Alzheimer's disease

Overlapping Conditions

PCOS and metabolic syndrome are overlapping conditions and share some of the same underlying physiologic abnormalities. Some women with PCOS display most of the criteria for the diagnosis of metabolic syndrome. Women with metabolic syndrome typically develop endocrine imbalances that can affect thyroid, ovarian, and reproductive function.

PCOS is associated with metabolic syndrome because insulin resistance, which affects glucose and fat metabolism, contributes to both conditions. Since PCOS is variable from woman to woman and can involve many interwoven imbalances, some women with PCOS may have such a pronounced degree of high blood pressure and cholesterol that metabolic syndrome is the primary diagnosis. Other women may display more of a hypothyroid tendency with reproductive hormone imbalances, so the concomitant diagnosis of metabolic syndrome is less applicable. These two conditions are like overlapping Venn diagrams, with insulin resistance in the shared area.

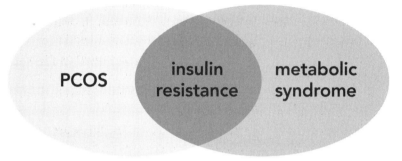

Genetic Predisposition and Lifestyle Factors

There is a strong familial occurrence of metabolic syndrome, especially in racial groups prone to the condition, such as those from the Indian subcontinent or individuals of African, Hispanic, and American Indian descent, indicating a genetic predisposition to the condition. The cause of metabolic syndrome, however, is multifactorial, and a polygenetic (involving many different genes) nature to the syndrome is emerging. Lifestyle factors, such as excessive consumption of refined carbohydrates and fats and lack of exercise, also contribute to the development of metabolic syndrome.

Refined Carbohydrates

A "refined" carbohydrate refers to a carbohydrate-based food that has been processed in such a way as to strip it of some of its original fiber and bulk to produce a more "refined" product. Sugar cane is a whole food, but the table sugar that is processed out of sugar cane is a refined carbohydrate. Corn on the cob is a whole food high in carbohydrates, but the cornstarch and high-fructose corn syrup that are processed out of the corn are refined carbohydrates. Whole buckwheat kernels, whole wheat, and barley are high in fiber and complex carbohydrates, but when they have been milled into flour, some nutrients may be lost — and even more may be lost when the germ and bran are stripped from the grains.

Although refined carbohydrates contribute to metabolic syndrome, "whole" fruits and vegetables are good for us because they contain fiber and many beneficial, if not vital, nutrients. The recipes in this book aim to include lots of whole foods and very few refined carbohydrates.

Treatment for Metabolic Syndrome

The treatment for metabolic syndrome will depend on the individual presentation, but all patients will benefit from dietary therapy and exercise. Even a moderate reduction in overall calories to support weight loss can be beneficial. In addition to general calorie reduction, particular emphasis should be placed on avoiding foods with a high glycemic index (see page 79) and that contain processed and refined carbohydrates, as well as fats from animal and processed foods.

Nutrients and herbs that reduce insulin resistance are appropriate in all cases. These substances are listed in Part 2. If you have frank heart disease, blood clots, or hypertension, your physician might choose a more aggressive nutritional, herbal, or pharmaceutical course of therapy.

Dietary Measures to Reduce Metabolic Syndrome

1. Reduce or eliminate all simple sugars, refined carbohydrates, and high-sugar foods (such as candy, cookies, pastries).
2. Avoid soda pop and high-fructose corn sweeteners.
3. Reduce all processed carbohydrates and flour products.
4. Reduce animal fat and limit all fat.
5. Reduce all fried foods, hydrogenated oils, and margarine.

Chronic Obesity

Well over 50% of all women with PCOS, perhaps as high as 70%, struggle with their weight. The degree of obesity appears directly proportional to the level of elevated ovarian and adrenal androgens, including testosterone, and to the degree of insulin resistance. Conversely, weight loss correlates with an improvement in elevated hormones and blood sugar.

"Central obesity" refers to the accumulation of fat about the trunk or midsection and is associated with PCOS, diabetes, insulin resistance, and metabolic syndrome. In addition to the insulin resistance and elevated androgens seen with these conditions, women with PCOS also appear to display abnormalities with the hormonal signals that direct the storage and burning of fat.

Some of the most successful therapies for dropping the excess weight involve improving insulin sensitivity, reducing elevated androgens, adopting a low glycemic index diet, and exercising more. Improving hormonal balance will support weight-loss efforts, and losing weight will support hormonal balance in a mutually reciprocal way. Obviously, losing weight is one important approach to treating PCOS.

PCOS facts

Rapid Dietary Changes

Some evolutionary biologists have proposed that many genetic hormonal tendencies contributing to PCOS originate from a relatively rapid change from the pre-agrarian age diet to the current diet. Food has become much more readily available, and these biologists suggest that ancient genetic hormonal balances have not adjusted accordingly. Pre-agrarian humans had frequent food shortages, worked long hours to obtain what food they could, and ate very few refined foods — certainly not the sugar and corn syrup products stocked on the shelves of every convenience store today. The rapidly increasing rates of diabetes, heart disease, and PCOS coincide with the rapid changes in the modern human diet.

Elevated Androgens and Weight Gain

The elevated levels of androgens in PCOS promote the storage of nutrients and the buildup of body tissues, which make it difficult to lose weight. Postmenopausal weight gain and altered fat distribution are examples of how powerful hormonal changes can affect body weight and fat deposits. The postmenopausal fall of estrogen allows for a relative increase in androgens.

Leptins and Adipokines

Leptins are hormones that are involved with directing fat metabolism. And a group of cytokines, the adipokines, including adiponectin, are other compounds that direct fat metabolism. The levels of both leptins and adipokines may be abnormal in overweight women with PCOS.

A group of enzymes, the beta-steroid dehydrogenases, play a role in metabolizing steroids, and these enzymes have also been found to be abnormally increased in obese women with PCOS. Researchers in Denmark have proposed that elevated levels of these dehydrogenases can promote excessive cortisol (an adrenal hormone) in the peripheral fat cells and in the subsequently increased glucocorticoid activity. Elevated glucocorticoids are also associated with weight gain and fluid retention in women with PCOS.

Measuring Body Weight

There are several accepted methods for calculating a healthy weight.

Waist-to-Hip Ratio

While we do not need to achieve an hourglass waist to be healthy, the relationship between our waist and hip circumferences can be an indicator of our health.

The waist-to-hip ratio is calculated by measuring the circumference of your waist (the narrowest part of a lean person's torso), roughly 1 inch (2.5 cm) above the navel, and comparing it to the circumference of the widest part of the hips. Having a smaller waist-than-hip circumference is associated with health, fertility, and longevity. The ratio will be a number smaller than 1, such as 0.7 or 0.8. A reversal of those numbers (1, 1.5, 2, and so on) is associated with diabetes, cardiovascular disease, numerous other diseases, and a shortened life span.

Waist Circumference

The International Diabetes Federation has proposed specific waist circumference measurements to define central obesity — and, therefore, to determine the risk of developing diabetes and heart disease. A waist circumference of more than 32 inches (80 cm) is defined as central obesity and is also associated with metabolic syndrome. This number may vary slightly depending on the skeletal frame size and shape of a particular race or genetic body type. The "waist" is roughly midway between the crest of the hip bones and the bottom of the rib cage, typically 1 inch (2.5 cm) above the navel.

PCOS facts

Fertility and Body Mass Index

A lower body mass index (BMI) of 30 or less is associated with greater fertility than higher body mass indices. Some fertility specialists recommend achieving this BMI before using any fertilization drugs or technologies, such as in vitro fertilization. Because these technologies are invasive, expensive, and have low success rates, it seems logical to improve the BMI and to support hormonal balance through diet, exercise, and nutritional supplements first.

Body Mass Index

The body mass index, or BMI, is a measure of the height-to-weight proportionality of an individual. BMI is calculated using a simple mathematical formula, where your weight is divided by height squared: $pounds \div feet^2$ (or $kilograms \div meters^2$). For example, if you weigh 150 pounds (68 kg) and you are five foot eight (1.75 m), your BMI = 22.

BMI Interpretation

- BMI 18 to 25 is considered normal
- BMI 25 to 30 is considered overweight
- BMI over 30 is considered obese
- BMI over 40 is considered morbidly obese

BODY MASS INDEX TABLE

BMI	19	20	21	22	23	24	25	26	27	28	29	30	31	32	33	34	35	36
Height (inches)	Body Weight (pounds)																	
	NORMAL						OVERWEIGHT					OBESE						
58	91	96	100	105	110	115	119	124	129	134	138	143	148	153	158	162	167	172
59	94	99	104	109	114	119	124	128	133	138	143	148	153	158	163	168	173	178
60	97	102	107	112	118	123	128	133	138	143	148	153	158	163	168	174	179	184
61	100	106	111	116	122	127	132	137	143	148	153	158	164	169	174	180	185	190
62	104	109	115	120	126	131	136	142	147	153	158	164	169	175	180	186	191	196
63	107	113	118	124	130	135	141	146	152	158	163	169	175	180	186	191	197	203
64	110	116	122	128	134	140	145	151	157	163	169	174	180	186	192	197	204	209
65	114	120	126	132	138	144	150	156	162	168	174	180	186	192	198	204	210	216
66	118	124	130	136	142	148	155	161	167	173	179	186	192	198	204	210	216	223
67	121	127	134	140	146	153	159	166	172	178	185	191	198	204	211	217	223	230
68	125	131	138	144	151	158	164	171	177	184	190	197	203	210	216	223	230	236
69	128	135	142	149	155	162	169	176	182	189	196	203	209	216	223	230	236	243
70	132	139	146	153	160	167	174	181	188	195	202	209	216	222	229	236	243	250
71	136	143	150	157	165	172	179	186	193	200	208	215	222	229	236	243	250	257
72	140	147	154	162	169	177	184	191	199	206	213	221	228	235	242	250	258	265
73	144	151	159	166	174	182	189	197	204	212	219	227	235	242	250	257	265	272
74	148	155	163	171	179	186	194	202	210	218	225	233	241	249	256	264	272	280
75	152	160	168	176	184	192	200	208	216	224	232	240	248	256	264	272	279	287
76	156	164	172	180	189	197	205	213	221	230	238	246	254	263	271	279	287	295

Source: Adapted from *Clinical Guidelines on the Identification, Evaluation, and Treatment of Overweight and Obesity in Adults: The Evidence Report.*

Strategies for Losing Weight

Dietary therapy, nutrient supplements, herbs, and exercise are primary ways to help reduce insulin resistance, balance hormones, and lose weight. In turn, losing weight helps improve cellular response to insulin.

PCOS facts

The Rewards of Weight Control

As little as a 5% reduction of body weight has been shown to increase metabolic and hormonal regulation in women with PCOS. One study on obese 12- to 22-year-old females showed that weight loss alone was capable of restoring normal menstruation.

The numerous dietary, nutritional, and herbal therapies described in the following chapters will help make it easier for you to lose weight by improving your cellular responses to insulin, fat metabolism, and hormonal balance.

BODY MASS INDEX TABLE

BMI	37	38	39	40	41	42	43	44	45	46	47	48	49	50	51	52	53	54
Height (inches)	Body Weight (pounds)																	
	OBESE			EXTREME OBESITY														
58	177	181	186	191	196	201	205	210	215	220	224	229	234	239	244	248	253	258
59	183	188	193	198	203	208	212	217	222	227	232	237	242	247	252	257	262	267
60	189	194	199	204	209	215	220	225	230	235	240	245	250	255	261	266	271	276
61	195	201	206	211	217	222	227	232	238	243	248	254	259	264	269	275	280	285
62	202	207	213	218	224	229	235	240	246	251	256	262	267	273	278	284	289	295
63	208	214	220	225	231	237	242	248	254	259	265	270	278	282	287	293	299	304
64	215	221	227	232	238	244	250	256	262	267	273	279	285	291	296	302	308	314
65	222	228	234	240	246	252	258	264	270	276	282	288	294	300	306	312	318	324
66	229	235	241	247	253	260	266	272	278	284	291	297	303	309	315	322	328	334
67	236	242	249	255	261	268	274	280	287	293	299	306	312	319	325	331	338	344
68	243	249	256	262	269	276	282	289	295	302	308	315	322	328	335	341	348	354
69	250	257	263	270	277	284	291	297	304	311	318	324	331	338	345	351	358	365
70	257	264	271	278	285	292	299	306	313	320	327	334	341	348	355	362	369	376
71	265	272	279	286	293	301	308	315	322	329	338	343	351	358	365	372	379	386
72	272	279	287	294	302	309	316	324	331	338	346	353	361	368	375	383	390	397
73	280	288	295	302	310	318	325	333	340	348	355	363	371	378	386	393	401	408
74	287	295	303	311	319	326	334	342	350	358	365	373	381	389	396	404	412	420
75	295	303	311	319	327	335	343	351	359	367	375	383	391	399	407	415	423	431
76	304	312	320	328	336	344	353	361	369	377	385	394	402	410	418	426	435	443

Nutrients and Herbs

Natural agents that help reduce insulin resistance include chromium, inositol, prickly pear cactus, and legumes, among others. Of special value is *Serenoa repens* (saw palmetto), which is currently a popular treatment for men with prostatic enlargement because it reduces the overstimulating effects of too much testosterone on the hormone-sensitive prostate gland. Women may also benefit from using saw palmetto. Folkloric wisdom credits the small black ripe fruit of this tropical palm with reproductive hormone–balancing effects.

Q. What more can I do to help lose weight?

A. Exercise! Plan a way to work regular exercise into your daily routine. An exercise program can be as simple as taking regular brisk walks, dancing, or starting a weight-lifting routine. Use hand weights and ankle weights at home or while walking to help build muscle. Your muscle mass helps the body to burn fat. Even 10 minutes daily of using hand weights can promote muscle growth.

If you are up to joining a gym or participating in a community sports league, such as volleyball or soccer, it would be even better. But if time, money, and fitness level don't allow, there are plenty of ways to get more movement and activity into your day.

Walking is free. Just open your front door and do it! All you need is a sturdy pair of walking shoes. Consider walking around the block once or twice before you take your morning shower. Once you're ready for the next step, walk a mile or two before work or before getting started on the day's chores. Or if you have time, take a nice long walk to have breakfast or a cup of tea with a friend, and then walk back home.

Why not walk or bike instead of drive to do your errands? Could you walk to the market every day for that day's groceries instead of loading up the car once a week? If not, park in the farthest parking spot from the store — either across the lot or even blocks away. At the very least, don't seek out the closest parking spot to the stores you need to go to. Choose the lonely spots the farthest away from the door or perhaps even a few blocks away, and you will at least get a little bit more walking in on an errand day. Always take the stairs (not the elevator or escalator). Perhaps 10 minutes of stretching, 10 minutes of calisthenics, and a half-hour walk each evening after work or dinner would be manageable with your routine.

Sometimes people are more successful in sticking with an exercise routine when regular activities are planned with a friend or a group. You are much less likely to cancel or put off the activity (Oh, it's a little rainy today, I'm a little too busy today, and my back is a little stiff today…) if you have friends who are meeting you. Or consider becoming a "mall walker." In our rainy Pacific Northwest climate, a number of my female patients walk back and forth along the length of the local mall. Maybe you and your partner could have exercise dates — from a weekend hike to a weeknight dance date to a lively game of Twister with the kids.

You don't have to participate in sports to get exercise, and the possibilities are endless. A friend and I once blew up about 50 balloons using an air compressor. We tried, with our kids, to see how many balloons we could keep up in the air at once. I think the game went on well over 45 minutes while our dinner was in the oven.

A top-to-bottom cleaning of the house certainly counts as a non-sedentary activity! If it's a nice day, haul your wet laundry outside and hang it up to dry instead of using the dryer. Work in the garden. Repaint the hallway. Mow the lawn. Sweep the garage. You can get exercise and your chores done at the same time. If you pay someone to do your house cleaning, yard work, dog walking, or other chores so that you put in a few more hours at work, consider the health benefits you'll reap from doing those chores yourself. Aim to reduce sedentary activities and increase any and all types of activity. The more fun you have being active, the better.

Heart Disease

Many women with PCOS are at risk for cardiovascular disease, and those with the dual diagnosis of metabolic syndrome doubly so. Women with PCOS should be evaluated for cardiovascular disease, specifically for hyperlipidemia (high cholesterol) and hypertension (high blood pressure).

Hyperlipidemia

"Hyperlipidemia" refers to the condition of excess fat or lipids in the blood. Lipids, especially cholesterol and triglycerides, are elevated in PCOS and metabolic syndrome. Elevated blood lipids are known to induce changes in artery walls, in the expandable/contractible smooth muscles in the artery walls, and in the more delicate innermost cells, known as the endothelium, which line internal body cavities.

Lipid Tests

Two lipids, cholesterol and triglycerides, are commonly evaluated as part of routine physicals and health screening blood tests. However, several other lab tests, such as c-reactive protein and homocysteine, are two other indicators of the severity and urgency of the risk. These tests should be considered in women with PCOS, particularly when there is a family history of heart disease and high blood pressure.

Hypertension

Hypertension, or high blood pressure, exacerbates the cellular damage caused by hyperlipidemia. In turn, inflamed and damaged arteries increase the risk of heart attack, stroke, and blood clot formation. Smoking increases these risks even more.

Hypertension is extremely prevalent in older women with PCOS, particularly those who are obese. Again, insulin resistance is highly linked to this abnormality in women with PCOS. Heart disease is a major cause of death in all older women, but some researchers have found a seven-fold increase in heart attack risk in older women with PCOS compared to older women without PCOS. All women with PCOS should be evaluated for cardiovascular disease.

Thyroid Dysfunction

The thyroid gland helps control the basal metabolic rate in the body — how high the body temperature runs, how fast the heart beats, and how quickly foodstuffs are metabolized for energy. Having a combination of low thyroid function and low metabolic rate compounds problems of insulin resistance because the ability of cells to take up glucose and other fuels is already poor. This helps explain the relationship between thyroid function and insulin sensitivity and the abnormal elevations in lipids and glucose seen in both conditions.

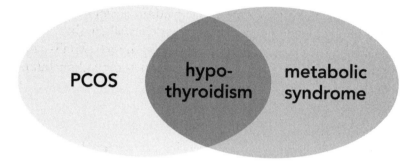

Metabolic Syndrome Association

Researchers report that women undergoing therapy to suppress excessive thyroid activity (hyperthyroidism) frequently develop metabolic syndrome — as quickly as 4 weeks following treatment. Hypothyroidism is also associated with elevations in insulin and insulin resistance.

PCOS facts

Prevalence

Thyroid dysfunction is more common in women with PCOS than in women without PCOS and is twice as common in women with diabetes than in women without diabetes. All of these research findings suggest that the health of the thyroid contributes to the risk of PCOS, diabetes, and metabolic syndrome. Abnormally low levels of thyroid hormones are associated with a higher body mass index, increased waist circumference, high blood pressure, and higher cholesterol and blood fats — all signs and symptoms shared by hypothyroidism and metabolic syndrome.

Greater Risk

Autoimmune thyroid disease is much higher in infertile women than in fertile women, and especially so in infertile women with PCOS. One study showed that women with PCOS were three times as likely to have autoimmune hypothyroidism compared to other women of similar reproductive age. Some women whose bodies are producing thyroid autoantibodies (antibodies to their own thyroid tissue) may actually have thyroid hormones in the normal range, but they may present with other classic symptoms of hypothyroidism, such as fatigue, constipation, central obesity, and chronic skin rashes. These symptoms may improve with a trial course of thyroid hormones.

Hypothyroidism

There are several different types of hypothyroidism, including autoimmune hypothyroidism and subclinical hypothyroidism. Specific blood tests, such as a peroxidase antibody test, can be performed to help distinguish between the various types of hypothyroidism.

Autoimmune Hypothyroidism

In autoimmune diseases, the body's immune system essentially attacks itself, with white blood cells producing antibodies to combat the believed threat in the body. In the case of autoimmune hypothyroidism, the white blood cells produce antibodies that attack the thyroid cells, causing inflammation and eventually leading to the destruction of thyroid tissue. Women with PCOS are more likely to be diagnosed with autoimmune hypothyroidism.

In one type of hypothyroidism, the body produces antibodies that attach directly to thyroid cells, causing inflammation and eventually leading to the destruction of thyroid tissue.

One way our white blood cells combat pathogenic bacteria and viruses is by producing antibodies against them. When the body produces antibodies against itself, in this case against the thyroid gland or against specific thyroid enzymes, the immune system is attacking its own body. There is a group of such diseases known as autoimmune diseases because the immune response is inappropriate and directed against the person, rather than an external pathogen. Women with PCOS may frequently be diagnosed as having autoimmune hypothyroidism.

Subclinical Hypothyroidism

The condition of subclinical hypothyroidism refers to a suspicion of poor thyroid function based on clinical symptoms; the hypothyroidism diagnosis, however, can't be confirmed by laboratory tests. Subclinical hypothyroidism may present with normal levels of thyroid hormones in the blood, yet results may show an elevated level of thyrotrophin-stimulating hormone (TSH), suggesting that the pituitary is working very hard to stimulate the thyroid to produce adequate amounts of thyroid hormone or that the thyroid gland is responding poorly to TSH.

Abnormally elevated TSH is associated with metabolic syndrome and PCOS as well as with hypothyroidism. Therefore, slightly elevated levels of TSH — even when circulating thyroid hormones are in the normal range — may be a significant finding. While some physicians may dismiss a slightly elevated TSH in a woman with otherwise normal thyroid function tests, others may connect the dots and interpret the slight elevation in TSH, combined with obesity, or menstrual irregularities, or infertility, or slightly high blood sugar, or combinations of other symptoms, as signs of PCOS. In such cases, natural and/or pharmaceutical thyroid support may improve PCOS and related issues.

Thyroiditis

Thyroiditis is an inflammation of the thyroid. It could be caused by infection or inadequate levels of iodine, or because of the autoimmune response of antibodies attacking the gland. Autoimmune thyroiditis is associated with some cases of PCOS.

Fertility

Thyroid hormones directly affect the ovaries, and they interact with prolactin and pituitary hormones. Thyroid hormones also contribute to the health of eggs in women's ovaries, and to sperm and sperm motility in men. There are, in fact, binding sites for thyroid hormones on human eggs, and there is a direct correlation between thyroid disease and negative pregnancy outcomes. Low thyroid function is one contributor to miscarriage, premature labor, and problem pregnancies.

PCOS facts

Inflammation

Inflammation of the thyroid occurs more commonly in adolescent girls with PCOS than in other adolescent females. In fact, close to 30% of young women with PCOS have been found to have thyroid antibodies, and more than 40% have been found to have thyroid abnormalities when tested with ultrasound. Recently, elevated adipokines, which are immune molecules released from fat cells, have also been associated with autoimmune thyroiditis.

PCOS facts

Thyroid Imbalance and Miscarriage

Women with PCOS who are struggling with infertility but having no success with clomiphene citrate therapy to stimulate ovulation have been found to have a higher incidence of thyroid imbalance than women with PCOS who respond well to clomiphene. Autoimmune thyroid disease is also associated with an increased risk of miscarriage in the first trimester. This is so common, in fact, that many fertility specialists recommend hypothyroidism testing for women with PCOS who are considering fertility drugs and/or are undergoing in vitro fertilization. In some cases, specialists may recommend thyroid medications as a preventative measure against miscarriage and as a supportive measure.

Treatments

The medication metformin and the medicinal herb *Commiphora mukul* (guggul) are effective in regulating thyroid hormones. Iodine and selenium are also used for this purpose.

Metformin

Metformin may help women with PCOS because — in addition to improving insulin resistance — the drug has been shown to have beneficial effects on altered thyroid function. Irregular results in thyroid function tests, particularly those that show autoimmune markers, such as antithyroglobulin and antithyroid peroxidase antibodies, are especially prevalent in those PCOS cases involving a significant degree of overlapping metabolic syndrome.

Q. What evidence is there of the effectiveness of metformin for thyroid disease?

A. Clinical trials on women with PCOS have shown metformin to reduce elevated TSH from the pituitary, suggesting that thyroid function has improved and/or the gland's response to TSH has improved, although it is also possible that metformin simply has toxic effects on the pituitary. In general, the higher the TSH level, the higher the body mass index, the higher the testosterone level, and the greater the degree of insulin resistance in women with PCOS.

Another study dosed women with the dual diagnoses of both PCOS and hypothyroidism with metformin or placebo for 6 months and ran thyroid function tests at the start and the completion of the half-year trial. Significant decreases in the elevated TSH were seen in the group receiving the metformin but not the group receiving the placebo.

This is not to say that all women with hypothyroidism should be on metformin. Natural medicines, whenever appropriate and effective, may also support healthy thyroid function and improve insulin response.

Guggul Treatment for Hypothyroidism

Guggul is the common name for the *Commiphora mukul* plant, a gummy, resin-yielding tree of the Burseraceae family, related to myrrh. Guggul has been used for obesity and high cholesterol in India for generations. Modern research suggests it may enhance thyroid hormone activity. Animal studies show that guggul reduces the effects of thyroid suppressive drugs. Steroidal substances in guggul gum increase the thyroid gland's uptake of iodine (iodine is needed to synthesize thyroid hormones). Guggul also enhances the activity of thyroid enzymes, which also supports the production of thyroid hormones. Both actions serve to improve thyroid hormone production.

Some studies suggest that guggul can metabolize fat, lower cholesterol, and lower blood sugar. The steroidal substances in *Commiphora mukul* are referred to as guggulsterones, and they have been shown to act on bile acid receptors in the liver in a manner that may help the organ process lipids and contribute to the hypolipidemic effect (and recent research suggests that they may also act on the intracellular nuclear receptors that are involved with basic cellular metabolic functions, including cholesterol metabolism, contributing to the plant's hypolipidemic effect).

Iodine

Iodine is a component of thyroid hormones, and optimal thyroid function depends on receiving a certain range of iodine in the body. It has been shown that both too little and too much iodine can suppress the thyroid gland or, less often, overstimulate the thyroid. Some of the richest sources of iodine are seaweeds and animal products, such as milk, fish, and eggs. Vegans may have a low intake of iodine and are most at risk for iodine deficiencies.

The thyroid gland takes up iodine and combines it with tyrosine to synthesize thyroxine, which is then converted to triiodothyronine, the active thyroid hormone. Although small doses of iodine (in the range of micrograms) appear to stimulate thyroid function, large doses of iodine (in the range of 500 milligrams per day) will, in some cases, inhibit thyroid function. In some cases, even as little as 3 milligrams per day may inhibit thyroid function. Ongoing iodine deficiency will typically result in goiter (enlargement of the thyroid gland) and low thyroid function.

The World Health Organization uses the term "iodine deficiency disorder" and estimates that more than 800 million people are affected and at risk of health problems due to inadequate iodine intake. When iodine is not available in the body to produce thyroid hormones, high levels of TSH result, which leads to free radical formation and may relate to some of the many inflammatory conditions of subclinical hypothyroidism and thyroiditis. This oxidative stress is likely to be seen in combination with selenium deficiency.

Iodine deficiency during gestation can cause abnormal brain and endocrine development in the offspring. In iodine-deficient areas of the world, iodine supplementation during pregnancy is recommended. On the other hand, excessive intake of iodine during pregnancy is known to lead to transient hypothyroidism in newborns. Maternal consumption of more than 2 or 3 milligrams of iodine per day is associated with the most severe thyroid suppression. The current recommendation for pregnant women is 150 to 220 micrograms per day. Although it is important to take a multivitamin that contains the recommended daily allowance for iodine, do not supplement iodine above this dosage without a physician's guidance.

Selenium

All of the iodinase and peroxidase enzymes (the enzymes involved in thyroid hormone production and regulation) are selenium dependent. Selenium and iodine work synergistically. Selenium is required to both synthesize and metabolize thyroid hormones and the iodinase enzymes needed to synthesize them. Selenium can affect iodine metabolism, homeostasis, and bioavailability. Selenium at a dosage of 200 micrograms per day may reduce thyroid antibodies in adults with autoimmune thyroid disease. One clinical trial of 169 pregnant women with hypothyroidism or subclinical hypothyroidism and with the presence of autoantibodies to the thyroid gland reported that selenium supplementation improved postpartum thyroid function.

Selenium is safe and non-toxic when taken at the recommended dose of 400 micrograms per day or less. It is credited with many antioxidant effects and may be added to the list of possible nutritional supplements for women with PCOS, especially those with hypothyroidism or subclinical hypothyroidism.

Thyroid Function and Anti-inflammatory Fats

Fat cells are one important source of certain compounds that mediate inflammatory responses in the body. One of these grouped molecules is called adipokines. At times, these compounds can be appropriate and needed; at other times, such as with PCOS, these compounds can be inappropriate and excessive.

Q. Is thyroid inflammation common in women with PCOS?

A. Yes. The high prevalence of thyroid inflammation in women with PCOS may be related to elevated inflammatory compounds, such as adipokines, in the body. Most women with PCOS have a greater number of fat cells, so a greater number of such inflammatory compounds is produced. Furthermore, the stimulus to produce these compounds may be greater in women with PCOS due to the many other abnormal hormonal signals. It is somewhat of a chicken-and-egg scenario: having low thyroid function may promote or aggravate insulin resistance and inflammatory responses, and having insulin resistance may lead to the accumulation of fat cells, which produce inflammatory substances that impair thyroid function.

The risk of developing ovarian cancer is two or even three times higher in women with PCOS. Similarly, women with PCOS are three times more likely to develop endometrial cancer than other women. Some researchers have also reported a specific type of uterine cancer known as endometrial adenocarcinoma in women with PCOS. In women with amenorrhea, the lack of regular menstruation prolongs the stimulating effects of hormones on the endometrial lining and can lead to hyperplasia (excessive buildup) of the hormone-sensitive tissue, which in turn can progress to cancerous changes in the cells.

Ovarian and Endometrial Cancer

Many of the body's tissues are sensitive to hormonal levels. An obvious example would be the uterine lining (the endometrium), which builds up and sheds each month in relation to the rising and falling of hormone levels and the menstrual cycle. Other hormone-sensitive tissues include the breasts and the ovaries. Cancers of all these tissues are known to be promoted by excessive hormonal stimulation and a lack of balancing and protective hormones.

Q. Is it true that oral contraceptives reduce the risk of ovarian cancer?

A. Oral contraceptives have been shown to reduce the risk of ovarian cancer. Birth control pills (BCPs) are sometimes recommended as an ovarian cancer preventive measure for women with PCOS, particularly for those who are obese. But some physicians have concerns that this recommendation is ill conceived and that a more holistic evaluation is needed, in particular to address the increased risks of other conditions. For example, oral contraceptives are associated with increased risk of blood clots and other cardiovascular risks, and they have been shown to *increase* insulin resistance. The use of BCPs in women with PCOS may also worsen glucose tolerance and contribute to metabolic dysfunction and risks. One study showed that women with metabolic syndrome who took BCPs suffered a worsening of glucose regulation and an increase in abdominal fat accumulation.

Q. What can I do to prevent and treat PCOS so that I don't get any of these associated diseases?

A. There is plenty you can do to help balance your hormones and manage PCOS. The following chapters will detail what foods to steer clear of in order to avoid straining your hormonal balance, and what nutrient-rich foods to enjoy that will help you regulate your hormones. The chapter on dietary therapies will give you lots of tools, recipes, and techniques to help you prepare delicious, nutritious food.

Specific nutritional supplements, such as vitamin D and chromium, can help support blood sugar regulation and cellular responses to insulin. And lesser known nutritional supplements such as *pinitol* and specific forms of inositol have also shown efficacy. Details and reasonable dosages are discussed in chapter 4.

Finally, herbal medicines can also support hormonal balance. There is a growing body of research validating folkloric uses of herbs to restore fertility, regulate menstrual cycles, and reestablish menses in cases of amenorrhea. Many herbs are proven to help balance blood sugar, reduce insulin resistance, lower elevated cholesterol, and protect artery walls from being damaged by high blood fats and sugars. Chapter 3 discusses the latest research on the efficacy and safety of herbs appropriate for managing PCOS.

Women with PCOS are at an increased risk for hormonal cancers due to long-time term hormonal imbalance and excessive stimulation of the hormone-sensitive tissues. High blood pressure, blood sugar imbalances, and nutritional deficiencies may also contribute to an increased risk. Obesity appears to increase the risk of ovarian cancer in women with PCOS more than any other individual contributor. Recently, insulin resistance has been added to the list as a strong risk factor for developing endometrial cancer. Balancing the body's hormones and (if obese) losing weight may help reduce the increased risk of cancer.

Part 2

Managing PCOS

Chapter 3

Dietary Therapy for PCOS

CASE HISTORY
❧ *Tina*

Tina was 60 years old when she first visited our clinic. She was married, with two children, and worked full time in the public school system. She is relatively tall at 5 foot 10 (1.77 m), large-boned, strong, and reasonably fit, but she had put on about 30 pounds in 30 years. Her job kept her seated most of the day, and when she got home in the evenings, she reported having little energy to do much but read the paper, prepare TV dinners for herself and her husband, straighten up the kitchen, and go to bed.

When I asked her about her diet, she replied, playfully, that she thought ketchup counted as a vegetable. She avoided salads and loved frozen meals because of their convenience. Pastries were a staple in her diet. She resisted cooking anything for herself from scratch. Her eating habits had become a problem, not only because Tina was a big lady, but also because her blood pressure and cholesterol levels were climbing. Pharmaceutical therapies were becoming increasingly less effective.

Tina came in to see me hoping to find a natural remedy for her high blood pressure and LDL ("bad" cholesterol) levels. When I reviewed her blood work, I noted her blood sugar to be on the far high end of the normal range. She had some side effects from the pharmaceuticals she was on and disliked the idea of increasing the dosage. The majority of older women with PCOS have trouble with high blood pressure, and often losing weight and improving hormonal balance will be of benefit.

Tina had a normal menarche and regular cycles for many years, but when she was ready to have children in her late 20s, she struggled with infertility and finally she and her husband resorted to in vitro techniques. She had one child via in vitro fertilization and adopted a second child after repeated attempts at pregnancy failed. Her menses stopped altogether in her early 40s, and while one physician blamed the amenorrhea on early menopause, I suspected that Tina's menses stopped due to the hormonal imbalances typical of PCOS. At this same time her blood pressure spiked and she began pharmaceutical blood pressure medications at the age of 35 and cholesterol medicine in her 50s. Her blood pressure was less responsive to these medicines over time, necessitating higher dosages and additional drugs to control.

We began by changing her eating habits to achieve a basic healthy diet and then added nutritional and herbal therapies for her PCOS. We began the long and gradual process of optimizing her diet to promote weight loss and hormonal balance. As we talked, it was apparent that Tina actually liked many healthy foods, she just didn't like cooking, washing the dishes, or shopping for healthy ingredients. At 60 years of age, we can be quite set in our ways, so I began to look for ways of improving Tina's nutrition that fit her habits. Since Tina was in the habit of thawing a frozen entrée before she left for work in the morning, and then putting it in the oven or microwave when she got home from work, we brainstormed on prepacking and even freezing some healthy bean loaves, salmon burgers, and casseroles that she should cook after work, as was her custom. We also devised some slow cooker recipes that she could make in the evening and set in the fridge overnight. In the morning she would put the ceramic pot into the crock pot, turn it on, and come home to hot soup or stew.

We discovered that the school staff lunch and break room was full of temptations. Her co-workers brought in cookies, boxes of doughnuts, and trays of brownies to share. This room was the hub of all school staff socializing. We discussed taking a walk outside the building for her lunches and breaks and avoiding setting foot in that room whenever possible. Tina found other staff and faculty with similar struggles and goals, and found buddies to pair up with for lunchtime walks, rain or shine.

Tina's retired husband, who did most of the grocery shopping, joined Tina in her diet and fitness program. He was very willing to shop for the ingredients and make a salad every day to add to our slow cooker and homemade dinner entrees. After dinner every night, Tina and her husband prepared a sack lunch of dinner leftovers for her to take to work in the morning. They went for a half-hour walk in the neighborhood before dinner each weeknight and much longer walks in local parks and trails each weekend.

Through the efforts of this gentle daily walking routine, herbal and nutritional supplements, and some significant dietary changes, Tina's cholesterol and blood pressure dropped and she lost some weight. Her risk of suffering a future stroke or heart attack declined in turn. We stopped the cholesterol drug she was taking and replaced it with natural alternatives. We also dropped her diuretic drug, which we suspected was robbing her of important minerals. After a year and a half she was able to get off her remaining blood pressure medication altogether. Her husband ended up losing a bit of weight as well. He had been very supportive for Tina, and instrumental in helping to implement the numerous dietary changes.

Dietary therapy is the number one strategy for managing PCOS and associated conditions. Some foods are simply not good to eat if you have PCOS, while other foods are therapeutic. Eliminating or avoiding problematic foods can be difficult because some may be your favorites. Any change in lifestyle is hard, but changing what you eat may be the hardest. Nobody wants to be deprived of enjoyable food items unless there are compelling reasons. We trust that the reasons we present in this chapter for adopting a new dietary program are certainly compelling, even lifesaving.

PCOS Dietary Program

- High complex carbohydrate foods
- Low glycemic index foods
- Whole foods
- High-fiber foods
- High-protein foods
- High essential fatty acid foods
- Therapeutic foods

PCOS Dietary Goals

1. Reduce total calories consumed to standard levels for your sex, age, and activity level.
2. Limit your intake of refined carbohydrates in favor of complex carbohydrates.
3. Eat carbohydrates that are lower on the glycemic index.
4. Avoid processed and refined foods and eat whole foods instead.
5. Increase fiber in your diet to improve glucose regulation.
6. Select lean meats, especially fish, and eat legumes to meet protein needs.
7. Avoid trans fats and increase foods rich in omega-3 essential fatty acids.
8. Increase intake of PCOS therapeutic foods.

Healthy Diet

Adopting a healthy diet can improve your hormonal balance and be a valuable treatment for PCOS. If you avoid challenging your blood sugar balance with large meals and high glycemic index foods, your body will be able to metabolize sugar and carbohydrates more efficiently. If you are able to consume more anti-PCOS nutrients, such as chromium, magnesium, and *D-chiro-inositol*, this too can help improve your core metabolism and support optimal hormonal balance. Weight loss and dietary improvements alone have been shown to help restore irregular menstrual cycles and improve fertility, blood pressure, cholesterol, and blood sugar — and decrease the risk of many of the diseases associated with PCOS.

Macro- and Micronutrients

The body needs a regular supply of energy, or calories, to maintain basal metabolism (the energy needed by the body at rest for breathing, blood circulation, and digestion) and to enable all other physical and mental activity. The food we eat provides that energy through three major nutrients, or macronutrients: carbohydrates, proteins, and fats. Food also contains micronutrients, chiefly minerals and vitamins, which enable the major metabolic reactions involving carbohydrates, proteins, and fats in the body. Micronutrients assist in digesting and absorbing macronutrients.

Digestion begins immediately after food enters the mouth, when it is exposed to various enzymes in the saliva, stomach, and small intestine. The digestive process breaks down whole macronutrients into smaller molecules, such as amino acids and fatty acids, which are then absorbed by the small intestine.

Food Groups

The United States Department of Agriculture (USDA) and Health Canada both publish food guides designed to improve your diet. These guides categorize food items into several food groups:

- Grains and legumes
- Vegetables and fruits
- Milk and dairy products
- Meats and meat alternatives
- Nuts and seeds

PCOS facts

Restoring Balance

In women with PCOS, the normal healthy balance of macronutrients in their diet has been disrupted. For example, an excessive consumption of simple carbohydrates can challenge blood sugar balance and optimal basal metabolic rate. When excessive caloric or carbohydrate consumption is combined with a deficient intake of important nutrients, hormonal and metabolic balances in the body can be further disrupted. Balancing the diet helps to restore the reproductive, hormonal, and metabolic functions of the body for women with PCOS. Restoring nutritional balance, along with metabolic and hormonal balance, is the key to managing PCOS.

(These tables have their pros and cons. There is still the need to be able to choose a quality grain, meat, and dairy product. For example, the use of quinoa as your grain in a salad is a "good" grain choice, while a pastry or other processed white flour food is a "bad" grain choice. A convenience store hot dog is a "bad" meat choice, while poached salmon is a "good" meat choice. And an ice cream sandwich is a "bad" dairy choice, while a bit of cottage cheese with your breakfast fruit is a "good" dairy choice. A person could make a number of "bad" food choices and still fulfill the dietary guidelines outline.)

USDA Food Guide

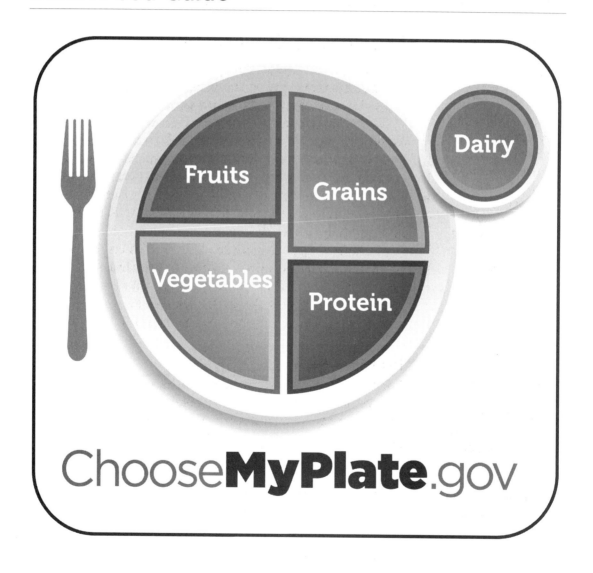

Eating Well with Canada's Food Guide

Recommended Number of *Food Guide Servings* per Day

	Children			Teens		Adults			
Age in Years	2-3	4-8	9-13	14-18		19-50		51+	
Sex	Girls and Boys			Females	Males	Females	Males	Females	Males
Vegetables and Fruit	4	5	6	7	8	7-8	8-10	7	7
Grain Products	3	4	6	6	7	6-7	8	6	7
Milk and Alternatives	2	2	3-4	3-4	3-4	2	2	3	3
Meat and Alternatives	1	1	1-2	2	3	2	3	2	3

What is One Food Guide Serving?
Look at the examples below.

Fresh, frozen or canned vegetables
125 mL (½ cup)

Bread
1 slice (35 g)

Bagel
½ bagel (45 g)

Milk or powdered milk (reconstituted)
250 mL (1 cup)

Cooked fish, shellfish, poultry, lean meat
75 g (2 ½ oz.)/125 mL (½ cup)

The chart above shows how many Food Guide Servings you need from each of the four food groups every day.

Having the amount and type of food recommended and following the tips in *Canada's Food Guide* will help:

- Meet your needs for vitamins, minerals and other nutrients.
- Reduce your risk of obesity, type 2 diabetes, heart disease, certain types of cancer and osteoporosis.
- Contribute to your overall health and vitality.

For the full guide, please contact Health Canada or visit their website (www.hc-sc.gc.ca).

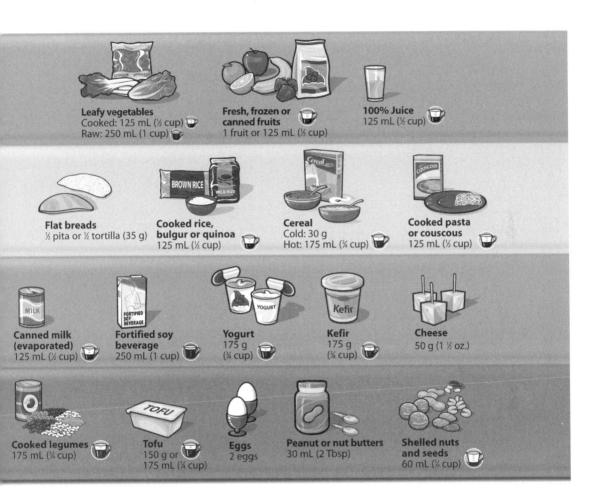

Leafy vegetables
Cooked: 125 mL (½ cup)
Raw: 250 mL (1 cup)

Fresh, frozen or canned fruits
1 fruit or 125 mL (½ cup)

100% Juice
125 mL (½ cup)

Flat breads
½ pita or ½ tortilla (35 g)

Cooked rice, bulgur or quinoa
125 mL (½ cup)

Cereal
Cold: 30 g
Hot: 175 mL (¾ cup)

Cooked pasta or couscous
125 mL (½ cup)

Canned milk (evaporated)
125 mL (½ cup)

Fortified soy beverage
250 mL (1 cup)

Yogurt
175 g
(¾ cup)

Kefir
175 g
(¾ cup)

Cheese
50 g (1 ½ oz.)

Cooked legumes
175 mL (¾ cup)

Tofu
150 g or
175 mL (¾ cup)

Eggs
2 eggs

Peanut or nut butters
30 mL (2 Tbsp)

Shelled nuts and seeds
60 mL (¼ cup)

Energy Balance and Weight Loss

Published food guides may specify the number and size of servings needed to receive adequate calories, which vary according to gender and age. For example, a moderately active 19- to 30-year-old woman should consume 2,000 to 2,200 calories daily. Food analysis calculators have been developed to determine the calorie content of most food items. These are available on the Internet and in print from a dietician.

If you consume more calories than your body "burns" from basal metabolism and physical activity, you will likely gain weight, because the excess calories are stored in the body as fat. This is a state of energy excess. If you burn more calories than you consume, an energy deficit can occur and you will likely lose weight as your body burns those calories stored in body fat. Once you achieve your desired weight, you can maintain that weight by balancing the calories you consume with the calories you burn.

Balanced Diet

Women with PCOS need to balance their calorie intake with their activity level to help manage their weight. They also need to eat balanced meals with servings from all food groups, but taking care to limit grains and grain products, especially those containing flour and processed grains and even more so those also containing any of the various sugars. This is an important consideration because not all foods in any one group are equally valuable in managing PCOS. The USDA MyPlate food guide uses a plate to show how much you should eat from each food group.

Most food guides recommend eating a balanced or proportioned diet of macronutrients, deriving 25% to 35% of your daily total calories from carbohydrates, 20% to 35% from proteins, and 20% to 30% from fats. Many experts also recommend aiming to ingest more than 25 grams of fiber each day and keeping your sodium intake well below 3 grams a day.

Nutrient Deficiency

Eating a greater proportion of carbohydrates in the diet, at the expense of protein, is detrimental to health, as is forgoing the quality carbohydrates and the required nutrients they contain and loading up on excess proteins. Favoring any one group – carbohydrates, proteins, or good fats — may lead to deficiencies in the nutrients that the minimized food group contains. For example, strict vegans and vegetarians need to take special care that they are getting all the protein and amino acids their bodies need from vegetable sources. People who live on chicken

Energy Balance

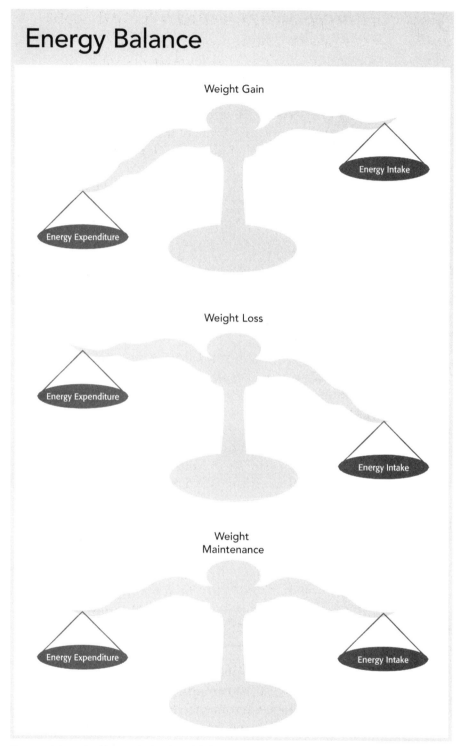

Weight Gain

Energy Intake

Energy Expenditure

Weight Loss

Energy Expenditure

Energy Intake

Weight
Maintenance

Energy Expenditure

Energy Intake

Source: Adapted with permission from McCrindle B. *Get a Healthy Weight for Your Child.*
Toronto: Robert Rose Inc., 2005.

and burgers may need to take care that they are covering
the nutritional basics, because meats do not provide the full
complement of vitamins and minerals needed.

Favoring one or two foods and eating them over and over can also lead to nutritional deficiencies that are easily avoided when you eat from a wide food "palette." For example, if you eat a "mono" diet of corn and few or no other vegetables, you can develop pellagra, a vitamin B3 deficiency. This disease was common in the American South when corn was the staple food. Better to rotate through as many different fresh fruits and vegetables as possible for optimal nutrition. It is also more interesting to have a variety of foods and nutrients to choose from.

Similarly, a steady diet of white bread lacks adequate nutrients to maintain good health. The milling process for white flour strips the grain of fiber and some essential nutrients. That's why flour mills fortify white flour with vitamin B1 (thiamin), vitamin B2 (riboflavin), vitamin B3 (niacin), and folic acid. Deficiencies in these vitamins can result, respectively, in beriberi, ariboflavinosis, pellagra, and spina bifida birth defects.

Complex Carbohydrates

Carbohydrates include fruits, vegetables, grains, and legumes. During the digestive process, they are broken down into sugars, or saccharides. Chief among these sugars is glucose. Other saccharides include sucrose (table sugar), fructose, dextrose, and maltose.

Glucose is the very first product generated by the photosynthetic process in plants. It is an extremely versatile and important molecule upon which the entire food chain is based. Plants transform glucose into other sugars, starches, and myriad higher compounds. All animals must ingest these sugars to sustain life.

There is a huge variance in the quality of the foodstuffs available to provide carbohydrates, and our choices can have a great impact on our health and particularly on PCOS, diabetes, and metabolic syndrome. We can obtain carbohydrates from a variety of different food groups, including whole grains, fruits, and vegetables. Grains typically provide fiber, B vitamins, vitamin E, and trace minerals, as long as they are not milled and refined. The colorful fruits and veggies contain numerous essential antioxidant nutrients along with simple sugars and complex carbohydrates and a good deal of fiber. Legumes are high in protein, fiber, and *pinitol* in addition to providing carbohydrate macronutrients. Creating your diet from a balanced combination of these carbohydrate sources can best help provide a diverse array of important vitamins, minerals, and other nutrients. Avoid eating only grains and no fruits or vegetables, but also only fruits and no whole grains. By eating from all these groups we will best cover our nutritional needs.

Q. What is the difference between refined and complex carbohydrates?

A. Refined carbohydrates are foods, most often grains, that have been milled and processed in such a way as to concentrate the sugars and simple carbohydrates, often discarding the fiber and valuable nutrients with them. Refined or simple may be more appealing to some people. For example, white bread is softer and spongier than whole-grain breads. However, in addition to being stripped of many important nutrients, refined and simple carbohydrates break down much faster in the digestive process than complex carbohydrates, spiking blood sugar levels to a greater extent than complex carbohydrates.

Complex carbohydrates occur naturally in whole grains, fruit, and vegetables and break down more slowly than refined carbohydrates. They provide a slow and gradual rise in blood sugars, whereas sugars from refined carbohydrates will cause the blood sugar to spike.

Sugar requires insulin to enter cells. Reducing your intake of refined carbohydrates can reduce the sugar load in the body and improve insulin sensitivity. Carbohydrates also contribute every bit as much to the accumulation of fat in the body as eating fat itself. Studies have shown that eating a low refined carbohydrate diet can help you lose more weight than an indiscriminate calorie-restricted diet.

Safe Sweetener

To avoid high-calorie sweeteners, such as sucrose (table sugar) and high-fructose corn syrup, without sacrificing flavor, try using *Stevia rebaudiana*. The sweetness of stevia is not due to simple sugars, but rather to compounds known as glycosides (including steviosides, steviolbiosides, dulcosides, and rebaudiosides). Stevioside is said to be 200 times sweeter than table sugar. Stevia has a caloric and glycemic value of

Soft Drink Dangers

Consumption of soda pop and other sugar-laden fruit drinks and punches is associated with an increased risk of obesity for all women. A study on the prevalence of obesity in California reported that those who drink soda are 15% more likely to be obese than people who drink no soda. Those who drink 1 or more sodas every day are 27% more likely to be obese than those who drink no soda. To avoid fructose sugars in soft drinks, consider buying a juicer and making your own fresh fruit and vegetable juices. See the beverages listed in the Recipes section of this book for other ways to satisfy your thirst and taste buds without consuming refined sugars and high-fructose corn sweeteners.

zero. It promotes little or no insulin response. Interestingly, the Coca-Cola Company has funded research on stevia to isolate the sweet-tasting substances, and the work has been published in the journal *Molecules*.

Sneaky Simple Sugars

Q. How do I know if a food item contains simple or refined sugars?

A. The average consumption of processed sugars has increased dramatically with each generation for the past several hundred years. Today, sucrose (common table sugar) and other simple sugars can comprise as much as 15% of the whole diet, and that number is much higher for some people. The use of high-fructose corn syrup has also increased significantly in the past generation. A single can of soda pop may have 10 teaspoons (50 mL) of sugar in it, often in the form of high-fructose corn syrup. Some sources have estimated the annual consumption of high-fructose corn syrup per person to be well over 60 pounds (27.2 kg). In an attempt to avoid using the word "sugar" on the ingredient list of a product label, some manufacturers will instead use one of a long list of synonyms. Watch out for these words because they are in fact simple refined sugars:

- Dextrin, dextrose, maltodextrin
- Malt, barley malt, maltose
- Corn syrup, corn sweetener
- Evaporated cane juice
- Fructose, high-fructose corn syrup
- Invert sugar, raw sugar, turbinado sugar, cane sugar
- Lactose, xylose, sucrose, saccharose
- Rice syrup
- Agave nectar

Glycemic Index

The glycemic index is a measure of how quickly carbohydrates are broken down into simple sugars during digestion and how quickly those sugars are absorbed into the bloodstream. The glycemic index is determined by ingesting a precise quantity of a single food, one that delivers 50 grams of carbohydrates, and then testing the blood sugar levels several times over the following 2 or 3 hours.

The complexity of the carbohydrate affects the pace at which sugars are teased out of the fiber. Foods that cause a large and rapid increase in blood sugar are considered to be high on the glycemic index. Foods that raise the blood sugar to a lesser degree are low on the glycemic index.

Most carbohydrate food items have been ranked on a glycemic index. Each food item is given a numerical value relative to 100, the glycemic value of pure glucose. For example, sucrose (table sugar) is valued at 65 on the glycemic index, and fructose is valued at 19. In general, processed breads, cereals, sugar, candy, and sweetened drinks are high on the glycemic index, and whole fruits, vegetables, beans, and nuts are low on the glycemic index.

PCOS facts

Symptom Reduction with Low GI Foods

Studies have shown that diets with a low glycemic load can help reduce PCOS symptoms. General dietary goals for PCOS should include reducing total caloric intake and reducing the intake of foods high on the glycemic index.

Glycemic Index of Common Foods

Glucose: 100
High glycemic index: 70 and higher
Moderate glycemic index: 50 to 70
Low glycemic index: below 50

Food Group / Item	Glycemic Index
Sweeteners	
Corn syrup	100
Table sugar (sucrose)	85
Rice syrup	65
Honey	54
Agave nectar	30
Pure maple syrup	19
Fructose	10
Stevia	0
Grains, Breads, Cereals	
GRAINS	
White rice	90
Instant rice	86
Wild rice	81
Whole corn kernels	78
Oatmeal	77
Millet	71
Cornmeal	70
Bulgur wheat	67
Couscous	65
Brown rice	55
Buckwheat	54
Whole wheat	48

Food Group / Item	Glycemic Index
Whole amaranth	35
Whole quinoa	35
Whole rye	35
Sprouted wheat	25
Whole barley	25
Sprouted barley	15
BREADS	
Rice bread	100
Cooked cornmeal/ polenta	98
Taco shells	97
Baguettes	95
Corn tortillas	78
Doughnuts	76
Croissants	70
White bread	70
Whole wheat bread	69
Burger buns and hot dog buns	67
Pancakes	67
Kamut bread	54
Quinoa bread (60% quinoa flour)	50
Rye bread	50
Sprouted grain bread	45
Whole-grain pumpernickel	45
Pasta, whole-grain	44
Pumpernickel	40

Food Group / Item	Glycemic Index
Quinoa flour	40
Sprouted grain breads	35
Wheat germ	15
CEREALS	
Instant oats	92
Puffed rice	85
Corn flakes cereal	83
Crisp rice cereal	82
Cheerios	74
Grape-Nuts	67
Oat bran	15
GRAIN SNACKS	
Rice cakes	84
Soda crackers	74
Corn chips	72
Rye crisp crackers	67
Popcorn	55

Nuts and Seeds

Food Group / Item	Glycemic Index
Chestnuts	60
Peanut butter	40
Tahini	40
Sesame seeds	35
Sunflower seeds	35
Cashews	24
Almonds	15
Hazelnuts (filberts)	15
Pine nuts	15

Food Group / Item	Glycemic Index
Pistachios	14
Peanuts	14
Sprouted seeds	14
Walnuts	14

Legumes and Beans

Food Group / Item	Glycemic Index
Fava beans	50
Split peas	45
Canned refried beans	38
Adzuki beans	35
Black beans	35
Hummus	35
White beans	35
Chickpeas	33
Kidney beans	32
Sprouted lentils	30
Lentils	29
Mung beans	25
Soybeans	18
Bean sprouts	15
Carob powder	15
Green beans	15
Tempeh	15
Tofu	15

Food Group / Item	Glycemic Index	Food Group / Item	Glycemic Index
Vegetables		Eggplants	15
Potatoes, baked	100	Green beans	15
Potatoes, boiled	84	Lettuce	15
Carrots, cooked	80	Mushrooms	15
Squash	75	Olives	15
Rutabagas	72	All pickles	15
Beets, cooked	64	Radishes	15
Pumpkin	64	Sauerkraut	15
Corn	55	Snow peas	15
Sweet potatoes	54	Spinach	15
Parsnips	52	Summer squash	15
Yams	51	Tomatoes	15
Peas	44	Zucchini	15
Coconut	35	Avocados	10
Tomato sauce	35	**Fruits**	
Carrots, raw	30	Watermelons	90
Beets, raw	30	Dates	70
Bean sprouts	25	Pineapples	66
Artichokes	15	Raisins	64
Arugula	15	Canned fruit in syrup	60
Asparagus	15	Apricots	57
Bell peppers	15	Strawberries	56
Broccoli	15	Mangos	55
Cauliflower	15	Papayas	55
Celery	15	Bananas	52
Chile peppers	15	Persimmons	51
Cucumbers	15	Grapes	50

Food Group / Item	Glycemic Index
Oranges	46
Plums	42
Apples	39
Most dried fruits	36
Nectarines	35
Passion fruit	35
Pears	35
Pomegranates	35
Stewed apples, applesauce	35
Tangerines	35
Peaches	30
Blackberries	28
Blueberries	25
Gooseberries	25
Grapefruit	25
Raspberries	25
Cherries	25
Rhubarb	22

Dairy Products and Alternatives

Rice milk	84
Coconut milk	40
Soy milk	36
Chocolate milk	34
Low-fat fruit yogurt	33
Skim milk	32
Almond milk	30

Food Group / Item	Glycemic Index
Cottage cheese	30
Oat milk	30
Whole milk	27

Beverages

Beer	110
Soda pop	80
Mango juice	55
Cranberry juice (unsweetened)	50
Orange juice (unsweetened)	45
Grapefruit juice	45
Carrot juice	40
Tomato juice	35
Drinks prepared using half water and half juice	20
Water	0
Herbal teas	0

Condiments

Raw garlic	30
Dark chocolate	25
Tamari	20
Lemon juice	20
Pesto	15
Gingerroot	15
Culinary spices	5
Vinegar	5

How to Use the Glycemic Index

Eating foods low on the glycemic index, especially when fiber and legumes are included, has been shown to improve glucose control in women with PCOS and diabetes.

1. **Aim to eat 5 to 10 different whole fresh fruits, vegetables, and legumes each day.** If you fill up on low GI foods, you will naturally eat fewer bread products, simple sugars, and processed foods, which not only have a higher glycemic value but also contain less fiber, fewer nutrients, and — in many cases — poorer-quality fats.

2. **Avoid a diet that consists predominantly of the foods highest on the glycemic index** — sugar, bread, rice, and potatoes, for example — especially at the exclusion of low GI fresh fruits and vegetables.

3. **Substitute foods high on the glycemic index with foods lower on the GI.** For example, eat boiled green beans (with a GI of 15) instead of boiled potatoes (with a GI of 100) with your dinner.

4. **Increase your fiber intake.** Fiber helps slow the digestion of carbohydrates and improves insulin resistance. If you love a food high on the glycemic index, take care not to consume it often and aim to eat only a small portion of it combined with high-fiber foods that reduce the glycemic load.

5. **Eat legumes to lower the high GI foods in your meals.** Legumes are low on the GI and contain an impressive amount of fiber and good-quality protein, which can serve to blunt the glycemic load. Saponins found in legumes and beans have been shown to lower elevated blood glucose and cholesterol. Legumes also contain *pinitol*, a relative of *D-chiro-inositol*, noted for improving insulin resistance. Many clinical trials have shown that legumes can benefit people with diabetes, anyone with high cholesterol, and those with hormonal imbalances, such as PCOS.

6. **Avoid overeating foods high on the glycemic index.** The GI of a food can be tempered by the quantity consumed. For example, a piece of candy might have a very high glycemic index, but eating just one little piece (not that we are encouraging it) won't result in a high glycemic load on the body. But if you are having two pieces of white toast, jam, hash brown potatoes, and a sugar- or corn syrup–sweetened fruit drink for breakfast, you are putting a high glycemic load on the body and the blood sugar will remain high for several hours as your body works to process the large amount of high glycemic index foods.

7. **Evaluate the whole meal, rather than individual food items,** to make sure you are preparing meals that won't spike your blood sugars.

8. **With the glycemic index in hand, see how the ingredients in the recipes in this book are generally low on the GI.**

Glycemic Index Limitations

Glycemic values have some limitations: the index calculations are not exact because the behavior of foods in different individuals can vary, and judging the diet by glycemic index alone does not give the whole picture.

Glycemic Load

Some authorities believe that the glycemic load (GL) is a more useful measure of food value than the glycemic index alone. The GL is a number calculated by using the glycemic index of a food and the amount of carbohydrate in that food: GL = GI x carbohydrate (grams) ÷ 100.

For example, the glycemic index of a ripe banana is 51 and the amount of carbohydrate in it is 25 grams: 51 x 25 ÷ 100 = 12.75. This number can be rounded up to 13. In another example, an orange has a glycemic index of 43 and contains 11 grams of carbohydrate: 43 x 11 ÷ 100 = 4.73 (round up to 5). Therefore, the orange will have a smaller impact than the banana on the systems in the body that maintain normal blood sugar control.

Cooking

Glycemic index rankings are affected by how foods are cooked. Cooked carrots have a much higher glycemic index than raw carrots because cooking breaks down the fiber, and the glucose can be absorbed much more quickly. Cooking grains, beans, and vegetables for a long period of time will increase the glycemic index because the fiber, which otherwise slows the digestion of starches and sugars, is broken down. Cooking with a bit of salt or vinegar may lower the glycemic index of many vegetables because this causes many molecules, not just the sugars, to be broken down, which results in trapping some of the starches in complex structures that are digested more slowly.

Calculation Variations

Due to the various ways that the glycemic index can be calculated, sometimes the glycemic index figures for a given food differ in the literature. Part of this has to do with the test subjects chosen to gauge blood sugar responses, and sometimes figures vary from morning to afternoon to evening. For some people, a food consumed in the morning on an empty stomach will spike the blood sugar more than the same food eaten later in the day after breakfast has already been digested. Those with good blood sugar control in general will show less of a spike in blood sugar than someone with poor blood sugar control.

Fat Content

There are some very unhealthy fried and fatty foods that have low glycemic values. This is because fat lowers the glycemic index. High-fat foods may appear falsely healthy in terms of glycemic index alone (look at the figures for rice cakes compared to potato chips, for example). Beware of food advertisers manipulating the glycemic index to sell their junk foods.

Whole Foods

Paying attention to glycemic values encourages people to avoid foods that are unhealthy in general, so-called junk foods, and to favor eating more whole fruits, vegetables, and legumes. You want to avoid empty calories, poor-quality fats, and foods lacking much redeeming nutritional value. Opting for whole fresh fruits and vegetables over anything canned, boxed, or otherwise processed will yield a lower glycemic index to the whole day's diet — better than any diet that involves opening cans, boxes, wrappers, packages, or fast-food bags.

At least 50% — if not 75% — of your diet should be whole foods. Whole foods include fruits, vegetables, grains, mushrooms, nuts, and a variety of whole fresh spices, seaweeds, or even fresh fish and meat in their whole, unprocessed forms. For example, apple slices are a whole food, but apple juice is not.

Common Whole Grains

- Quinoa
- Barley
- Amaranth
- Brown rice
- Wild rice
- Corn
- Whole wheat
- Buckwheat
- Rye

Side Benefits of a Whole-Food Diet

For managing PCOS, it is more important to avoid the empty calorie, fat-laden, processed carbohydrates than it is to be a slave to avoiding the higher glycemic index foods. In addition, whole fruits and vegetables, with a few exceptions like avocados and coconut, provide next to no saturated fat. If you are growing and purchasing whole organic fruits and vegetables, your synthetic chemical exposure and toxic load may be considerably less than that of people eating chemical-laden fast and processed foods.

Misleading Labeling

Q. Why do my favorite bagels say "Whole Grains" when it is obvious they were made from flour, not whole grain?

A. Whole-grain foods contain the entire kernel of wheat, or rye, or quinoa in its natural state, simmered in water, or soaked and sprouted into something soft and edible.

The commercial practice of adding the phrase "whole grain" to labeling has led to some confusion. When breads, bagels, muffins, pizza crust, and crackers are labeled "whole grain," it means that the entire grain is included in the flour and that the bran and germ were not removed. Although this is definitely superior to white bread that has been processed to remove the bran and germ, it is still flour and not actually a "whole grain." Some so-called whole-grain bread products may use 50% or more white flour and then throw in a bit of whole-grain flour so that they can legally use the term on the label.

In the recipes in this book, we have endeavored to use actual whole grains and to enrich or fortify recipes using flaxseed meal, brewer's yeast, oat bran, buckwheat, maca powder, and other healthy ingredients in order to reduce their glucose level and increase their fiber and nutrient content.

Weaning from Processed Grains and Breads

Q. If women with PCOS, metabolic syndrome, and insulin resistance should limit their consumption of carbohydrates and milled grains, why are there recipes using flour in this book?

A. If we were to advise you not to eat any bread, chips, or pasta, and instead only include 50 vegetable recipes in this book, we wouldn't really be giving you tools that you could work with or a realistic dietary approach that you could stick to in the long term. We included healthy grain and baked good recipes in this book so that it would be possible for people to give up the more harmful breads, snack foods, potatoes, and pastas. The expectation is that the higher-carbohydrate bread and muffin recipes in this book would always be paired with a bean spread, a vegetable soup, a raw salad, a steamed vegetable, or a vegetable casserole — a combination that would calculate into a meal with a low glycemic index. In this way, you can get your carbohydrate "fix," yet still reap the benefits of the diet plan.

Whole Versus Processed Grains

Grinding grains into flour causes them to behave more like sugar. Milling grain into flour generates heat, and heat reduces the healthy natural fats that are in grains. And if that ground grain is then sifted to remove the more fibrous bran and germ to yield the finest-textured flour, much of the fiber, chromium, and other nutrients in the grain will also be lost.

Any food that has been powdered will age and oxidize more rapidly. Once a food is sliced, peeled, chopped, or, in the case of grains, milled, the faster it will age and the more rapidly the nutrients will be lost. The smaller the particle size, the more exposed the surface area — and the more rapid the nutrient degeneration will be. Many commercially available flours have been milled in large industrial, heat-generating machines, sometimes refined, and they are typically packaged, shipped, and shelved in stores and warehouses — all contributing to a reduction in nutritional value.

Eating Habits

How we eat can be as important as what we eat. Eating quickly puts stress on insulin management; slowing down our eating habits will slow down the digestion process and help control insulin resistance.

Fast Foods

The story goes that the word "sandwich" comes from the card-playing habits of John Montagu, the 4th Earl of Sandwich, an 18th-century English aristocrat, while he ruled the Sandwich Isles. The earl loved playing cards and games with his friends — so much so that he was reluctant to take time away to eat when he was hungry. He invented the sandwich as something he could put together "fast" and eat easily with one hand while he continued playing cards. In our fast-food culture, many people don't bother with the fuss of cooking and eating a proper meal; rather, many would rather pull up to the drive-through and pick up their food, with one hand, and continue on their way. Unfortunately, these fast foods tend to be high in refined carbohydrates, high in poor-quality fats, and very low in fiber and quality nutrients.

Slow Foods

In response to the health issues resulting from fast-food culture, the "slow-food movement" has developed and recommends taking the time to prepare high-quality, healthy food. Paying attention to our food has physical, emotional, and spiritual value. Preparing nutritious food for yourself and your family results in good physical health. Cooking with others and enjoying meals together leads to emotional health. Maintaining an organic garden supports community and environmental health. Connecting to your garden and the cycle of the seasons brings spiritual health. Putting just an hour of effort into your food each day provides you with more than just the nutrients your body needs.

Cooking Grains

It is possible to add a bit of boiled barley, cooked quinoa, or another cooked grain — even cooked beans — to replace flour in many baked good recipes. Experiment to find your favorite flavors.

PCOS facts

Intact

Leaving grains whole and intact, rather than grinding them into flour, preserves their air-sensitive nutrients, quality oils, and fiber, which are all compromised or destroyed in the milling process.

Grind Your Own

Q. Can I grind my own flour like I grind my coffee?

A. If you grind your own fresh grains in small batches for immediate use, and you do not sift or refine them, the nutritional profile of your homemade product is likely to be much better than store-bought commercial flours — even the best of them.

A variety of different grinding apparatus exist for grinding small batches of grain. Electric semi-professional stone grinders would be on the higher end for those who love cooking and baking and wish to make grinding flour a habit. Some of the best commercial blenders will also work for small quantities. Metal-burred hand-cranked grinders that clamp onto the edge of a table or counter are also easy to use, although the process may be a bit more time-consuming and the flour may need to be run through twice. (Cooked beans can also be easily mashed in these hand-operated units.)

When traveling in other countries, I have frequently seen women using their hands to grind various grains and foods between two large river rocks, or pounding a large pestle up and down on top of foods in the deep well of a hand-carved wooden mortar, or tending homemade bamboo watermills. It is expected that grinding grains will take a bit of time and effort and needs to be done almost every day to give us this day our daily bread. Be it rice in Asia, corn and potatoes in South America, or wheat in North America, carbohydrate staples have been part of the diet in many cultures for generations.

Whole grains can be cooked in quantity at the start of the week, if desired, and stored in the refrigerator to use in quick salads, casseroles, and soups. In general, the whole grains can be prepared by simmering 1 cup (250 mL) of whole grain in 3 cups (750 mL) water until soft. To check for doneness, remove a small sample from the boiling water and taste it. If it is still hard or chewy, simmer for 10 more minutes and test again. Use a mesh strainer to drain.

Mixing Whole Grains

1. Mix wheat flour with ground flax, maca, and quinoa to yield fairly nutritious flour. The flour may be the least nutritious aspect of your recipe if you add applesauce, grated carrots, cooked pumpkin, banana purée, walnuts, chopped onions, minced hot peppers, blueberries, cranberries, molasses, wheat germ, and oat bran to the bread or muffins. You can create some very healthy bread and grain products at home.

2. Make only as much as needed for a single muffin, cracker, or bread recipe and work to add as many nutritionally redeeming ingredients to that recipe as possible.

3. If you absolutely love bread, consider purchasing a home grain mill to make your own fresh flour.

PCOS facts

Storing Whole Grains

To get the most nutrition out of your grains, buy small quantities and keep them whole and stored in your refrigerator (if you don't have the space, you can store them in a cool, dark cupboard).

Whole Foods Refuse

Like the grain and germ from whole grains, the pits, stems, cores, and otherwise commonly discarded parts of fruits and vegetables have many valuable nutrients. One way to use these nutrients is to keep a compost pile and, once composted, introduce these nutrients back to your garden beds. Another way to take advantage of the refuse from chopped fruits and veggies is to store them in a container in your refrigerator and — every few days — prepare a soup base with them by simmering the scraps in a stockpot or even a slow cooker. After 2 or 3 hours, strain and save the liquid for that night's dinner or save it for another day; make sure to use the vegetable stock within a few days — for soup or as the water in which you cook whole grains. The spent peelings can still be added to the compost pile.

Raw Foods

Raw food enthusiasts point to some of the research on advanced glycation (the result of the bonding of a protein or lipid molecule with a sugar molecule) produced by cooking foods as one of many reasons to eat more raw foods. Advanced glycation products result from roasting and searing foods and are believed to contribute to inflammatory and other disease processes in the body. Cooking foods destroys many enzymes and breaks down some of the more heat-sensitive vitamins, such as vitamin C. Frying foods adds to the fat content of the meal. Barbecuing or roasting foods also promotes the formation of cancer-forming agents in many meats.

How to Increase Raw and Lightly Cooked Foods in Your Diet

1. If adopting a raw food diet feels a little extreme for you, consider eating at least one raw food item, such as a raw fruit or a fresh salad, at every meal.

2. Raw foods need not be entirely cold, a prospect that can be unappealing in the middle of the winter in a colder climate. For soups in winter, purée raw vegetables in a blender to make a soup and then heat gently until pleasantly warm, remove from the heat, and serve promptly.

3. Try poaching or steaming your food in water, rather than frying in oil or roasting and barbecuing.

4. Steam broccoli, green beans, and other fresh raw vegetables for the shortest possible time, and at the lowest possible temperature, until just barely tender. Do not overcook vegetables.

Whole Foods Daily Menu Sample

Here is a sample menu for a day of whole-food meals, divided into servings and percentages. Try to make whole foods — vegetables, beans, and grains — comprise 75% of your food intake at each meal.

Whole-Food Breakfast (per serving)
- Whole raw fruit and nuts 75%
- Yogurt 25%

Whole-Food Lunch (per serving)

- Lentils, chopped tomatoes, chopped onion, chopped celery, chopped carrots, spices, and water 75%
- Quality baked good 25%

Whole-Food Dinner (per serving)

- Steamed broccoli 25%
- Raw salad of grated carrots, beets, slivered greens, kidney beans, garlic, vinegar, and flax oil 25%
- Whole cooked quinoa with onions, mushrooms, and steamed cabbage 20%
- Creamy avocado curry dressing 5%
- Poached garlic trout 25%

Meal Planning for Whole Foods

1. Aim to serve as many whole foods as possible in a meal.
2. Use both raw and cooked whole fruits, vegetables, and grains as the bulk of the diet.
3. Prepare a variety of cooked whole grains and beans every 3 or 4 days and store them in the refrigerator. At mealtime, combine these staples with raw and steamed whole vegetables.
4. Prepare one cooked whole food, one raw salad, and a few fruit slices for meals each day, or even for each meal.
5. Keep a variety of your favorite quality sauces and condiments on hand.
6. Add fish, chicken, tofu, and nuts to round out a meal and increase protein.
7. Eat mixed nuts instead of peanut butter.
8. Use fresh chopped tomatoes instead of a jar or can of tomato sauce.
9. Eat whole boiled wheat berries instead of wheat bread, whole fresh corn on the cob instead of cornmeal, and avoid corn syrup.
10. Increase whole food cooking by going to the organic market and choosing the best produce.
11. Choose a whole-food to be the main component of every meal. It is so simple to bake a squash, steam a head of broccoli, or roast ears of corn.

Serving Common Whole Foods

Beets: Grate and include in salads; simmer chunks in water or roast in the oven for a simple side dish; purée steamed or roasted beets for a beautiful soup base. Keep a whole cooked beet or two on hand, chilled in the refrigerator, to slice for snacks or to serve as the basis of cold lunch plates.

Broccoli: Eat raw, with a dip; eat raw in a salad; steam and eat plain (steam extra to store in a marinade); use the tougher stalks, boiled and puréed, for a soup base.

Carrots: Cut into long, thin strips for snacking and to eat with dips; cut into chunks and roast; cut into thin slices and stir-fry; grate or chop to eat raw in salads; use grated carrots with other grated and minced veggies in a dish of scrambled eggs.

Cauliflower: Eat raw, with a dip; eat raw in a salad; steam and eat plain (steam extra to store in a marinade); gently simmer the entire cauliflower head, positioned in a pan with an inch (2.5 cm) of water, and serve with a sauce poured over top; purée after steaming and use as a mashed potato substitute or as a layer in pasta-free lasagna-like recipes.

Celery: Cut into long, thin strips for snacking and to eat with dips; cut into thin slices and stir-fry; slice to eat raw in salads; steam until soft and purée for an unusual soup base; serve sliced stalks with homemade nut milk and toasted nuts and butters.

Corn: Because of its high glycemic index, corn is best combined with less starchy foods and other veggies; steam whole on the cob, cut kernels from the cob, and put them in a salad; roast whole cobs on a grill or under an oven broiler.

Cucumbers: Eat raw (does not cook well) in salads; cut into long, thin lengths for dipping in sauces; use a round as a cracker substitute for other spreads and minced veggies; combine finely chopped cucumber with yogurt and dill to make a side salad or a topping for lentil burgers and falafels.

Mushrooms: Bake portobello mushrooms filled with sauces; slice shiitake mushrooms and use in stir-fries; sauté any mushroom as a side dish; eat button mushrooms raw or briefly steamed and then marinated for storage in the fridge.

Onions and garlic: Use as a key ingredient in any soup, salad, casserole, or stir-fry; roast in the oven to sweeten; coarsely chop and then purée in a blender for the base of a creamy soup or salad dressing.

Radishes: Cut off the tips and set out in a little bowl for snacking; slice thinly for salads; carve into "flowers" for attractive edible garnishes.

Super-greens: Swiss chard, spinach, kale, collards, mustard greens, and bok choy can be thinly chopped to eat raw or can be "cooked" in lemon juice; steam and serve as a side dish; dehydrate until crispy and eat like chips; use whole large green leaves — grilled, roasted, or water-sautéed in a frying pan — as wraps for a variety of fillings.

Tomatoes: Chop for salads; slice to use with dips; use as a base for quick homemade sauces; include in a quick breakfast of stir-fried eggs and veggies or huevos rancheros; cut into rounds and use with cucumber slices instead of crackers when preparing hors d'oeuvres and snack foods.

Zucchini: Eat raw; grate into salads; sauté, roast, or grill as a side dish; grate zucchini and mix with eggs to make veggie hash browns; use in baked goods; slice a large zucchini in half, scoop out seeds, fill with lentils and onions or another filling, and bake until soft.

Squash: Cut lengthwise, remove the seeds, place flesh down on a baking sheet, bake until soft; purée or mash by hand to use as a soup base; add slightly under-baked squash pieces to stir-fries and casseroles; peel, seed, cut into chunks, and roast with onions and root vegetables in the fall.

Turnips and parsnips: Eat raw slices for a snack with hummus or another dip; grate turnips and use raw in salads or in veggie hash browns; chop into small chunks to include in soups, stews, and stir-fries; roast turnip for a surprisingly sweet side dish.

PCOS facts

No Potato, Yes Yam

Potatoes are not recommended in this diet due to their high glycemic index. The same goes for sweet potatoes. However, yams have a significantly lower glycemic index than potatoes. Grate yams to make hash browns; cut into chunks and bake in the oven for a side dish; cut into thin rounds and bake on a baking sheet for an alternative to chips. Simmer in water until soft and purée for mashed potatoes; use to prepare dumplings, breakfast patties, and baked goods.

High-Fiber Foods

A high fiber intake is recommended in all meals to help slow the release of sugars into the bloodstream and to blunt the glucose curve. Pectin fibers and guar gum, for example, have been shown to have a positive effect on blood sugar control. Pectin is found in the cell walls of all types of fruits and vegetables. Guar gum is a fiber extracted from algae and seaweed and is commonly used in the food industry as a thickener and stabilizing agent. One study found that consuming from 14 to 26 grams of guar gum per day resulted in a lowered insulin requirement and that a reduced amount of sugar spilled over into the urine.

You will naturally ingest a lot of fiber if you follow a diet that is high in whole fruits and vegetables. Aim to consume at least 5 — if not 6 to 10 — different whole, unprocessed fruits and (especially) vegetables each day.

High-Fiber Seeds and Meal

Plantago seeds, or psyllium (the basis for Metamucil), and *Linum* seeds (flax) help control blood glucose and blood lipids by slowing down digestion in the stomach and trapping some sugars and fats in the fiber bolus. Including these seeds or seed meals will enhance the nutritional profile and fiber content of a recipe and lower the glycemic index of the food. High-fiber oat bran and wheat germ act in a similar fashion.

PCOS facts

High Complex Carb, High Fiber Diet for People with Diabetes

The American Diabetes Association and the American Dietetic Association both recommend a diet that is high in complex carbohydrates, high in fiber, and low in saturated trans fat. This diet recommends that 70% to 75% of calories come from complex carbohydrates (whole vegetables, fruits, and grains), 15% to 20% come from protein, and 5% to 10% come from fat — all combined with 15 to 20 grams of fiber a day. The carbohydrate portion of this dietary regimen is high-quality complex carbohydrates (not flours, breads, or refined vegetable or cereal grain starches). Although this diet is stringent, it is effective in managing insulin levels in PCOS patients and people with diabetes.

High-Protein Foods

Proteins behave quite differently in the body than do carbohydrates. For one, protein is built from amino acids rather than from sugars. Although it is possible to convert protein into starch and fat for storage, the natural tendency is for protein to help repair and regenerate protein-rich tissues in the body, such as the muscles. Eating protein does not immediately contribute to the glycemic index of the meal. Meats, fish, dairy products, and eggs are high-protein foods, as well as nuts and legumes, both of which are recommended for women with PCOS.

Meal Planning with Protein

1. Aim to include protein of some sort in all of your meals, especially breakfast.

2. Don't skip breakfast, and especially don't eat a sugary breakfast. A sugary breakfast can get your insulin going and lead to unbalanced glucose control the entire day. Eating a solid breakfast with protein may also help reduce snacking and overeating later in the day. Make a smoothie, prepare hard-boiled eggs, heat up leftover soup, or have some nuts and fresh fruit. Legumes in the breakfast lineup have been shown to be particularly beneficial.

3. Take care not to ingest too much fat with the protein. Avoid fried meats, such as fried chicken, fatty bacon, and fast-food burgers, as well as processed, chemical-laden lunch meats.

4. Eat lean fish or hormone-free chicken in small amounts and combine the protein with plenty of vegetables.

5. Enjoy eggs. Eggs are a good source of protein and have nutritional content. They are especially healthy when poached or hard-boiled. Eggs may also be scrambled with lots of fresh vegetables, such as broccoli, carrots, and cauliflower — not just a few onions and tomatoes.

6. Include more beans in your diet. Beans and legumes have high fiber and protein content. Try huevos rancheros for breakfast, a lunchtime salad topped with kidney beans, or vegetable-lentil soup for dinner.

Essential Fatty Acid–Containing Foods

Fats are more calorie dense than a similar weight of carbohydrate or protein. Eating even a small amount can result in a high calorie load. The liver has to work hard to emulsify and process fats. An overworked liver is less able to process sugar, hormones, chemicals, and toxins. Women with PCOS who are looking to manage their weight need to control not only the amount of fat they eat, but also the kind of fat.

Q. What is a fatty acid?

A. Fatty acids are a component of animal and vegetable fats, and like glucose, are used as a fuel source in many tissues, particularly the heart and muscle. There are many specific types of fatty acids, and while the consumption of excessive fat in general is harmful, we do in fact benefit from the consumption of certain fatty acids, such as those found in whole grains, whole nuts and seeds, and fish.

> ### *Kinds of Fats*
>
> 1. Saturated fats
> 2. Trans fats
> 3. Unsaturated fats:
>   - Monounsaturated fats
>   - Polyunsaturated fats:
>   * *Omega-3 fatty acids*
>   * *Omega-6 fatty acids*

Kinds of Fat

There are three basic kinds of fat: saturated, unsaturated and trans fat. Fruits, vegetables, nuts, seeds, meat, eggs, and dairy typically contain a mix of the different kinds of saturated and unsaturated fat, while trans fats are mostly man-made and occur in processed foods, occurring very rarely in nature. Most foods contain a mix of the different kinds of fat. Olive oil, for example, contains about 75% monounsaturated fat, with about 25% polyunsaturated and saturated fat.

1. Saturated Fats

These fats can raise levels of low-density lipoprotein (LDL), or "bad" cholesterol, and have been linked to an increased risk for heart disease and cancers of the breast, colon, prostate, and pancreas. Of significance to PCOS patients: a high intake of saturated fat appears to increase insulin resistance.

Sources: Butter, cream, full-fat cheese, whole milk, fatty meats, and chicken skin. A few plant foods, such as palm, avocado, and coconut oil, are also high in saturated fat.

2. Trans Fatty Acids

These fats do not generally occur in nature and are manufactured by "partially hydrogenating" vegetable oils, a process that makes them more stable and solid at room temperatures. Trans fats are unhealthy and increase the risk of heart disease. They promote inflammation, raise LDL ("bad" cholesterol), and lower HDL ("good" cholesterol). Of significance to PCOS patients, trans fats can trigger heart disease and insulin resistance.

Sources: Foods made with partially hydrogenated vegetable oil (some cookies, cakes, crackers, pie crusts, and other baked goods) and margarine.

3. Unsaturated Fatty Acids

There are two kinds of unsaturated fats. Both have been credited for preventing disease.

Monounsaturated Fatty Acids

These fats do not raise LDL but they do raise HDL, the good cholesterol. Of significance to PCOS patients, monounsaturated fatty acids are believed to promote greater insulin sensitivity.

Sources: Olive oil and canola oil are good sources, as well as avocados, almonds, cashews, peanuts, and sesame seeds.

Polyunsaturated Fatty Acids

Polyunsaturated fats are commonly abbreviated as "PUFAs." There are also two kinds of PUFAs that should be consumed regularly in the diet: omega-3 essential fatty acids (EFAs) and omega-6 EFAs. EFAs are "essential" in that, like most vitamins and minerals, the body is unable to synthesize them and we must ingest them in our diets.

Omega-3 Fatty Acids

Omega-3 EFAs include alpha-linolenic acid (ALA), eicosapentanoic acid (EPA), and docosahexaenoic acid (DHA).

ALA is an omega-3 fatty acid found in plants. ALA is critical to our survival.

Sources: Flaxseed or flaxseed oil, canola oil, walnuts, and chia. The tiny seeds in whole kiwi, berries, and other fruits are additional sources.

EPA has been shown to reduce the risk of heart disease, cancer, and diabetes, and it reduces the risk of insulin resistance in women with PCOS.

Sources: Fatty fish and fish oils: bluefish, salmon, sardines, trout, and tuna, plus their fish oil. Fish are high in EPA due to the algae they consume, and algae-based products are on the market as vegetarian sources of EPA. Infants thrive on EPA, and human breast milk also contains EPA.

DHA is the most prominent fatty acid in the brain. It has been shown to have an impact on intelligence and attention deficit hyperactivity disorder (ADHD) among children, and Alzheimer's disease and cancer among adults.

Sources: Fatty fish (bluefish, salmon, sardines, trout, and tuna), plus their fish oils.

Omega-6 Fatty Acids

The most common omega-6 fat in our diet is linoleic acid, which has been shown to help prevent heart disease. However, omega-6 fatty acids are the precursor to inflammatory compounds in the body. Omega-3 fatty acids are known to help balance the inflammatory effects of omega-6 fatty acids. When omega-3 fatty acids are deficient, the beneficial effects of omega-6 oils may be diminished. Because corn, canola, and soy oils are used widely in the production of commercial and processed foods, many people consume excessive amounts of omega-6 and an insufficient amount of omega-3 oils.

Sources: Olive, canola, corn, sesame, sunflower, soybean, and walnut oils, as well as most nuts, seeds, and whole grains. Omega-6 fatty acids are commercially available as evening primrose, flaxseed, borage, and currant oil. These oils can be used to prepare salad dressings, and in some cases of deficiency, omega-6 oils are prescribed as nutritional supplements. Omega-6 fatty acids are not heat stable and should not be used to fry foods.

Cooking Oils

Many beneficial EFAs are not very stable and can be damaged with prolonged storage and even brief heating. Prolonged heating of EFAs can generate lipid peroxides that have inflammatory effects. Saturated fats, such as coconut oil, walnut oil, and avocado oil, are more stable at higher temperatures. Use coconut oil in very small amounts for frying or for high-temperature cooking, and use the more delicate oils, such as olive, canola, and flaxseed oil, for making salad dressings. With a good-quality pan, you can also "fry" foods in just water and add the delicate essential fatty acid oils afterward so that they are never heated to high temperatures.

Cooking and AGEs

Advanced glycation end products (AGEs) form naturally when certain foods are cooked at high temperatures or are industrially processed. AGEs are formed when foods are fried, broiled, or roasted but not when prepared using water-based cooking methods (poaching, steaming, boiling, and stewing). Some of the growing enthusiasm for a raw foods diet has evolved as the damaging effects of AGEs become better known. Using the lowest possible temperatures and adding water to the fry pan

PCOS facts

Lauric Acid

Coconut oil contains lauric acid, which may actually benefit the heart even though it is a saturated fat. There are some reports that coconut oil can help you lose weight, but it is not recommended to ingest by the spoonful. Using coconut oil may support weight-loss efforts in women with PCOS because it is healthier than common cooking fats, such as corn oil and margarine. Lauric acid in coconut oil has been reported to reduce blood fats in animal diabetes studies.

AGEs Control

AGEs are believed to contribute to diabetes and insulin resistance in women with PCOS. A high-AGE diet in animals can lead to damage to the pancreas and kidneys and results in an overall shortened lifespan compared to animals fed a low-AGE diet. The American Diabetes Association reports the consumption of AGEs in the diet contributes to all diabetes-related pathologies. If you have PCOS, prepare your food in a way that does not encourage the formation of AGEs, and make sure to ingest foods with antioxidant nutrients. Cook foods at the lowest possible temperature, add water to frying and roasting pans, and limit your consumption of roasted and barbecued meats.

rather than oil may be a happy compromise when wishing to stir-fry fresh veggies.

Glycation, or glycosylation, involves the fusion of proteins in foods to sugars, such as glucose and fructose. Although these substances formed in the cooking process tend to smell and taste great, they may contribute to inflammatory processes in the body. When the blood sugar is already high, as with diabetes and insulin resistance, the consumption of glycation products may promote disease. Consuming antioxidant nutrients, such as vitamin C, vitamin E, and beta carotene, reduces the harmful effects of eating foods cooked at high temperatures.

How to Use Your Frying Pan

1. Avoid oil and butter for frying whenever possible.
2. When frying, use a few tablespoons (30 to 45 mL) or even 1 cup (250 mL) water to prepare your food. The amount of water will depend on the quantity of food in the pan.
3. Place your onions or veggies to be "fried" in the water and stir frequently, adding a bit more water as needed and as evaporation occurs.
4. Covering the pan with a lid may help shorten cooking time and thereby preserve more enzymes and nutrients in the veggies; this is akin to steaming or poaching.
5. Save your oil for the sauce or dressing to be added at the last moment or in the form of a dressing or sauce at serving time.

Superfoods for PCOS

Some foods are especially effective in restoring nutritional, metabolic, and hormonal balance in women with PCOS. Make them the centerpiece of your diet.

Flaxseed

Flax seeds contain good-quality essential fatty acids, and the seed coat is high in lignans, which are beneficial for managing heart disease, metabolic syndrome, type 2 diabetes, and elevated blood glucose and cholesterol levels. Flax lignans are also credited with many anticancer and hormonal balancing effects. The high fiber and gummy nature of flaxseed meal helps lowers the glycemic index of regular grain flours.

Legumes

Some sources recommend avoiding legumes due to their starch content, but it's hard to ignore all the benefits they provide: they are high in complex carbohydrates, fiber, and saponins. Saponins in legumes have been shown to lower both blood fats and sugar. Legumes are also high in magnesium and *pinitol* and *D-chiro-inositol*, substances of great value for insulin resistance and hormonal modulation in women with PCOS.

Legumes include green beans, lima beans, navy beans, cannellini (white kidney) beans, mung beans, kidney beans, adzuki beans, chickpeas, lentils, soybeans, peas, and black-eyed peas. You need not be bored eating the same beans over and over. Early in the season, during spring and early summer, fresh green beans are at their best. Later in the growing season, shell beans are more plentiful. Throughout the winter, dried beans are satisfying in chilies, stews, and bean pâtés.

Sprouted Legumes and Grains

Soaking legumes and grains begins the chemical processes associated with sprouting. The energy inside the beans is stored in the form of starch, fat, and protein, and during a long soak these compounds are converted into other nutritious compounds and enzymes. Sprouting improves the availability of single amino acids, which support digestion and absorption

Meal Planning with Legumes

1. Use shelled or dried cannellini (white kidney), pinto, and other beans in soups, casseroles, bean salads, bean spreads, and pâtés, and as side dishes.

2. If you cannot be in the kitchen simmering beans for several hours, cook legumes in a slow cooker. Cooked legumes can be prepared and stored in the refrigerator to later throw into salads, stir-fries, and quick dinners. Canned beans are another user-friendly option.

3. Purée beans and refried beans for use in hummus, bean dips and spreads, huevos rancheros, and nachos.

4. Use chickpea, pea, and soybean flour in baked goods. Soy flour must be used sparingly in yeasted bread recipes because it contains a number of unique enzymes that can interfere with yeast and the rising process in leavened breads. A typical two-loaf bread recipe will usually call for 8 cups (2 L) of flour, of which only ⅓ cup (75 mL) may be soy flour. Other sorts of legume flours, such as chickpea (garbanzo bean) flour, can be added more liberally. Cooked oatmeal, cooked brown or wild rice, and cooked polenta can also be used in this way.

5. Soak beans overnight. This can improve nutrient availability and shorten cooking time. Dried lima, black, red, soy, navy, and cannellini (white kidney) beans are best soaked overnight, while lentils and split peas do not require soaking.

6. To reduce the incidence of flatulence, pour off the soaking water, rinse with cold water, and then use fresh water for cooking. For extreme sensitivity, you can even bring beans to a gentle simmer for 10 minutes and drain off the water, and then return to the pan with fresh simmering water.

7. If you are pressed for time or forgot to soak the beans the night before, you can pour boiling water over the beans, let them stand for an hour, drain, and then cook with fresh water.

8. Substitute cooked and mashed beans for about one-quarter to one-third of the wheat and grain flour in any bread recipe. Substituting bean flour will improve the nutrient profile of the bread as well as lower the glycemic index. Using legume flours or cooked legumes will also decrease the total carbohydrate content, replacing it with a bit more protein.

of the nutrients. Levels of vitamin C, vitamin E, and B complex vitamins all increase with prolonged soaking. Studies have shown that 2 days of soaking is better than an overnight soak in terms of nutrient content. Many dried beans require at least 2 hours of gentle simmering to soften up.

Some of the healthiest breads with the lowest glycemic indices are sprouted grain breads. Sprouting grains also reduces the amount of phytic acid, which is an organic acid that occurs naturally in grains and is known to bind to minerals and reduce their availability to the body. In fact, it is possible to make delicious bread with no flour at all, using only freshly sprouted grains. Add some sesame seeds, chopped nuts, and flax meal for a scrumptious, nutritious loaf that is far superior to most breads on the market. Sprouted grain bread is available at many health food stores.

How to Sprout Grains

1. Put 1 cup (250 mL) raw sunflower seeds, wheat, barley berries, or other whole grains in a wide-mouthed canning jar. Cover with water.

2. Top the jar with a mesh cover, to allow for a bit of air exchange.

3. Let the grains soak for 12 hours.

4. Drain the water, rinse with fresh water, and drain again. Store in a dark cupboard.

5. Rinse grains at least twice a day — three times is better — until the first white sprout has emerged from the grain and is about $\frac{1}{4}$ inch (0.5 cm) long. Once the small sprouts are beginning to emerge, the grain is ready to use. You can use the sprouts in breads, casseroles, and other recipes.

6. If you prefer, dry the sprouted grains on a baking sheet in an oven set to 200°F (100°C), leaving the oven door slightly ajar to achieve a temperature of 150°F to 175°F (70°C to 80°C), if possible. Many ovens do not have the option for such a low temperature. (You could also use a commercial food dehydrator on Low.) The dried sprouted grain is then ground into flour. This flour is more nutritious and easier to digest than flour ground from plain grains. Whole corn kernels, lentils, and many grains may also be sprouted by the same process.

Q. I've heard that buckwheat has special health properties. Would it help my PCOS?

A. Buckwheat contains high levels of *D-chiro-inositol*, a substance that has been shown to help restore hormonal balance in women with PCOS, especially when combined with *pinitol*, which is found in legumes. Buckwheat is not a true grain. It is a member of the Polygonaceae family, the same family as rhubarb. Buckwheat is lower on the glycemic index than wheat, corn, rice, millet, and many other true grains. Buckwheat preparations have been used as a traditional medicine in China for diabetes, but the value of buckwheat is rather new to Western medicine. Several animal studies have shown improvements in blood glucose levels and insulin sensitivity when buckwheat is included in the diet.

Maca Powder

Maca (*Lepidium meyenii*) powder may help reduce blood sugar and cholesterol levels and restore hormonal balance in women with PCOS. Maca powder homogenizes readily into blender drinks. Simply place nut or soy milk in the blender with a few raw nuts, chunks of fresh ripe fruit, and a heaping tablespoon (15 mL) of maca powder and pulse. For a thicker blend, use yogurt instead of milk — perfect for pouring on top of oatmeal or a bowl of fruit. Maca powder can also be used as a substitute for some of the regular flour in preparing baked goods.

Nut Meals and Milks

Although nuts are high-fat foods, often averaging around 50% fat, the fat in nuts is a healthy unsaturated type of fat that is beneficial to consume in small quantities. This does not apply to oil-roasted nuts, only raw nuts. Use raw nuts whenever possible. When toasting is desired, toast only the quantity needed immediately, and toast for the shortest time and at the lowest temperature possible to obtain the texture and flavor desired. Nuts can also be ground into an oily, granular meal referred to as nut meal. To help preserve the good fats in nuts, buy them in small quantities and store them in the refrigerator or freezer, if you have the room. Almonds, cashews, walnuts, and hazelnuts all contain beneficial oils and are versatile in the kitchen. One study on walnuts showed that they improved insulin response, adiponectin, and sex hormone–binding globulin levels. Eating almonds is also suggested to reduce elevated androgens.

Menu Planning with Nuts

1. Add nuts to smoothies and use as a garnish on salads, oatmeal, and fruit.

2. Grind nuts using a coffee grinder or a small, inexpensive hand-operated nut and spice grinder. Use the nut meal as a flour substitute in baked goods and desserts.

3. Make only as much nut meal as you need for your recipe. The good oils are better stored in whole nuts (the good fats will oxidize more quickly when ground).

4. Soak nuts in water to make nut milks. Almonds are one of the least expensive nuts and make excellent nut milk. Although cashews and pecans are a bit more expensive, they too make delicious nut milks to use in breakfast drinks and cooking. To make nut milk, pour boiling hot water over nuts, let stand for several hours or overnight, and then grind the mixture of water and plumped and softened nuts in a blender. Strain the liquid to remove the pulp, then enjoy as a nut milk drink. Make sure to reserve the pulp for use in baking, to mix with oatmeal, or to heat in a saucepan with other whole grains, dried fruits, or coconut to prepare fruit breakfasts and desserts.

Organic Foods

In addition to considering overall caloric intake, fat content, and glycemic value when preparing meals and snacks, aim for a diet that is as clean and chemical free as possible. Eating an organic diet that is free of hormones, pesticides, preservatives, artificial colors, and other chemicals will reduce the stress on your body, which must work to eliminate toxins. Studies have also shown that organic foods typically have a higher nutrient content than foods grown with industrial agriculture techniques.

Growth Hormones

Women with PCOS should be aware that many animal products may have a high hormone content. Bovine hormones are used to increase milk production and weight gain in cattle, and these hormones remain in the meat and milk and have hormonal effects in the body when we eat these foods. These ingested hormones can contribute to the hormonal load in our own bodies. Some American states allow the use of hormones in dairy cattle and some states have banned the use of hormones. Producers are not required to label hormone use, so purchase locally from milk and cheese producers you know don't use them.

Environmental Toxins

Pesticides, even though they are not hormones, are known to have hormonal effects in human tissue. Pesticides interfere with hormone synthesis, hormone release and storage, hormone transport around the body, hormone clearance from the body, hormone receptors, and thyroid function. Many environmental chemicals, including pesticides, are able to bind to estrogen receptors and disrupt reproductive and hormonal systems. Some of the man-made chemicals that we have flooded our planet and lives with are called "endocrine disruptors" due to the many ways that they interfere with normal endocrine and reproductive functions. Amphibians are being particularly affected because most live in chemical-laden rivers, streams, and wetlands.

Chemicals known as bisphenols are particularly associated with PCOS. Bisphenols are known to bind to estrogen receptors and are thought to contribute to inappropriate hormonal stimulation in the body. Because hormones are already abnormal and out of balance in PCOS patients, women with PCOS should avoid eating food contaminated with pesticides, eating organic foods as much as possible.

PCOS facts

Insulin-Like Hormones in Foods

One of the main hormones given to dairy cattle to increase milk production is insulin-like growth factor 1 (IGF-1). There are a few reports that claim that cows themselves develop a PCOS-like disease when given these hormones. Europe, Canada, New Zealand, Australia, and Japan have banned its use; American milk and cheese cannot legally be imported into these nations. The consumption of IGF-1 has been linked to hormonal cancers and other hormonal imbalances. Consumer advocate groups have complained for decades that U.S. labeling laws do not require dairies or producers to label clearly when a dairy product contains added hormones. Instead, consumers must do their own detective work.

The metabolic imbalances in women with PCOS may lessen their ability to tolerate IGF-1, and regular exposure to the hormone may contribute to cyst formation. Women with PCOS have been found to have higher levels of IGF-1 than other women.

Compliance

In this book, we have laid out a dietary program to manage your PCOS, but it is also important to address the emotional component to our relationship with food. If the dietary program in this book strips away many of your favorite foods, it is going to take some hard work to create a food program that you can enjoy — and you should be able to enjoy your food. It takes time to train children to appreciate vegetables, not just breads, sweets, and macaroni and cheese, but eventually they do. And you can take some comfort in knowing that, in time, you, too, will likely grow to appreciate other tastes and flavors.

If your favorite foods are grains, for example, search out recipes or experiment on your own to find or create a dish that has only a small amount of your favorite whole grain, such as bulgur wheat, brown rice, buckwheat, amaranth, or quinoa. Combine this with fresh vegetables and low-fat sauce. If you are saddened at the loss of your soda pop, find a high-quality unsweetened natural fruit juice (especially mixed with some prickly pear juice) and dilute it with a sparkling mineral water. Or if you are missing dessert, search for fruit dessert recipes. Eat whatever is ripe and delicious, in season, and looks good to you. Sprinkle a few raw nuts and cocoa nibs on fresh fruit slices. Put frozen banana slices in the blender with a little nut milk or coconut milk and fresh mango to make a dairy-free "ice cream" or smoothie.

Cookbook Surfing

Where can you find ideas for preparing nutritious and delicious meals to help manage PCOS? Get out all your cookbooks, including this one, and spread them out on the living room floor one evening or Sunday morning and come up with a week's worth of meals that will both keep you happy and satisfy the diet plan at the same time. Remind yourself of healthy forgotten favorites. Generate a shopping list and stock up on what you need. If you are having trouble getting motivated, make a menu plan and put it on the refrigerator door. Turn your kitchen into a fun place to be.

Kitchen Play

Clean the cupboards and organize things to make it easy on yourself. Get a new dish towel in your favorite color. Maybe buying a new floor mat or replacing the beat-up spatula will get you into the cooking mood. Turn on the radio or play your favorite CD in the kitchen. Put an orchid in the window. Get rid of all the bread, pasta, and any processed flour or sugar you have lying around. Toss out all the bad fats. Restock your kitchen with quality oils and nuts to use sparingly. Buy some stevia, agave nectar, honey, and molasses to use sparingly as sweeteners. Stock up on your favorite fruits and vegetables and place them in your clean and tidy fridge. Spend an hour once or twice a week cutting up onions and garlic and gingerroot so that they are handy and easy to use. Arm yourself with a complete collection of culinary spices and learn to use them. Being adept at seasoning foods with culinary spices can do wonders for your effort to eliminate fats, oils, and dairy-based sauces and dressings. If you can use gingerroot, fresh garlic, vinegars, freshly squeezed lemon juice, and spices, you won't even miss the cheese and the mayo and the commercial sauces and dressings. You might even enjoy growing a bit of mint, chives, or rosemary outside your kitchen door.

Q. I don't eat a very nutritious breakfast. What would you recommend that I do to change my breakfast eating habits?

A. The traditional American breakfast is not healthy for women with PCOS. Sugary cereals, coffee and doughnuts, bacon or sausage, toast and jam, pancakes and syrup all pose problems if you are trying to lose weight and manage your blood sugar levels.

If you can widen your concept of acceptable breakfast foods, you will be a lot better off. When I was traveling in Asia, I noticed most people ate a thin broth with rice and vegetables every morning. Could you eat soup for breakfast? How about dinner leftovers? Fruit and cheese? Beans and eggs? Quinoa and veggies? Or nut milk with fresh fruits and maca blended in? How about sautéed tofu, garlic, onions, and greens? Perhaps fish, cream cheese, grated carrots, and alfalfa sprouts on sprouted grain nut bread?

Sit down and make yourself a list of seven different recipes that you might enjoy and start replacing the "American" with the exotic. Aim to eat some sort of protein, such as fish, eggs, nuts, nut milk, or legumes, as this seems to help with blood sugar control for the rest of the day.

Many people say they are not hungry in the morning. Some people make the mistake of drinking coffee on an empty stomach and then deciding that they don't feel like breakfast after all. If you keep sipping coffee throughout the morning, your appetite can be suppressed for hours on end. Try holding off on the coffee until the breakfast is cooked, on your plate, and you are seated at the table. Eat first and you will find that you won't drink so much coffee.

If coffee is not the culprit, it could be that long-standing habits have suppressed the pattern of your stomach's acid production and your normal hunger levels. Many people find that if they make an effort to eat a small breakfast each morning, hungry or not, normal morning hunger returns in just a few days and they find themselves hungry upon waking in the morning.

The other common reason for skipping breakfast is that people are rushing to get to work on time, or to get the kids ready for school, and they don't have time to prepare anything. It's true; it can be very hard to find the time to squeeze cooking into the morning rush. There are a few options, however, that are so quick to prepare that they may work for busy people. Perhaps a quick smoothie prepared in the blender with soy milk, lecithin, some fresh fruit, a spoonful of maca powder, and fenugreek could be squeezed in. Slug it down and go. Or some quick scrambled eggs with vegetables left over from dinner.

Another option is to prepare some things ahead of time: hard-boiled eggs, poached fish, veggie hash browns, a quick cold plate. Prepare a container of chopped onions, garlic, mushrooms, chopped greens, and red bell pepper ahead of time to make preparing scrambled eggs or stir-fried tofu speedy. Bake a vegetable quiche when you have the time and simply heat a slice or two on the run in the morning. Bake two or three on a weekend or a free day and put two in the freezer for later. With just a little advance planning, it is not difficult to find a way to eat a nutritious breakfast.

Slow Eating

To complete your lifestyle change, aim to make your meals a time of slow-food self-nurturing. If you normally eat and run, make yourself set a place at table complete with tablecloth, full place setting, a candle and vase of flowers, and anything else that encourages you to relax and enjoy yourself. Serve yourself only a small serving to avoid the tendency to overeat. If you feel that you are still hungry after completing your plateful, first wait 10 minutes before going for a second helping, to give the food a chance to settle in your stomach. Eat slowly, thoroughly chew your food, and enjoy. These tips will help avoid overeating and they will foster appreciation for your food. Say a little prayer or give a little thanks for the food and earth from which your meal has come. This will help to make eating a very conscious act and help develop a sacred connection to your food and mealtimes.

Exercise

Lastly, find a way to include a bit of exercise into your mealtime routine. While in between steps of a recipe or while dinner is in the oven, sweep or scrub the floor or put on some music and dance like mad for 10 minutes. Use some hand weights and squeeze in 10 minutes of weight lifting. The greater your muscle mass and activity of the muscles, the more efficiently the muscles themselves can take up glucose, metabolize it, and help keep blood sugar low.

Many people find that once they start exercising, they naturally start trying to eat better. And once you've worked out, you won't want to waste all your good efforts by putting unhealthy foods back into the works.

Chapter 4

Nutritional Supplements for PCOS

CASE HISTORY

❧ *Starla*

When she first visited our clinic, Starla was 28 years old and employed full time in the retail industry. Starla's chief complaint was her weight. She was working out at a local gym, doing an aerobics class three times a week, and walking in her neighborhood on the weekends or anytime her schedule allowed — but she was frustrated to the point of tears that she had gained 2 more pounds (1 kg) the last time she checked.

Starla had fairly regular menses, but she would occasionally have cycles of 35 to 45 days in length once or twice a year, usually in the winter, but never in the summer. She also suffered from frequent itchy, eczema-like rashes, dry skin, and occasional constipation. Her fasting blood glucose was 98, near the top of the normal range. Her thyroid hormones were also in the normal range, but her thyroid-stimulating hormone (TSH) was in the high upper limit of normal. Although her lab work did not warrant the strict diagnosis of subclinical hypothyroidism, her symptoms combined with the big picture of her blood work suggested a less than optimal thyroid, metabolic, and reproductive hormone balance.

An effort was made to improve her metabolism using therapies appropriate to a more strict diagnosis of subclinical hypothyroidism. Starla was advised to take vitamin A and selenium supplements, as well as cod liver oil naturally containing vitamin D, all agents noted to improve skin complaints and support healthy thyroid and metabolic balance. We also began the herbal supplement *Commiphora mukul* in the form of a tincture at a dose of 1 teaspoon (5 mL) four times a day, and opuntia (prickly pear) "cocktails" prepared from 1 tablespoon (15 mL) of opuntia juice in a glass of sparkling mineral water with a citrus slice. We also sat down together and came up with a long list of legume recipes that she could incorporate into her diet on a daily basis.

Starla finally was able to lose some weight, starting about 10 weeks after beginning this routine. Her menses became more regular, and constipation improved promptly. Her chronic skin rash was last to improve, but it cleared in about 4 months' time. Follow-up blood work at 3 and 6 months showed that her TSH had returned to the middle of the normal range, and her fasting blood sugar dropped significantly, to 80 — just where I wanted to see it.

Starla's case is typical of women who suffer from the hormonal imbalances that typify PCOS, but due to the subtlety of the disorder cannot be diagnosed as having any specific condition based on lab tests alone. As physicians become more aware of the metabolic and hormonal disorders that contribute to PCOS, they are becoming more astute at recognizing the subtle presentations of PCOS. This is one reason why the statistics on the prevalence of PCOS goes up each year — physicians are recognizing PCOS symptoms more readily.

Starla could not be diagnosed, in the strictest sense, as being diabetic, hypothyroid, or with any specific reproductive pathology. However, the constellation of her many subtle symptoms were evidence of a metabolic dysfunction and an imbalance of reproductive hormones. It is obviously very frustrating for women like Starla to be told that everything is "normal" and to be sent on their way without receiving any help. On the contrary, there is a great deal that can be done to optimize metabolic function and hormonal balance for these women who fall through the cracks because none of their symptoms or lab tests are striking enough to fit in any "box" of established medical diagnoses.

Although the foods recommended in the PCOS dietary program are nutrient rich, there are a few nutrients so effective in managing PCOS that they should be taken as nutritional supplements. Nutrients include vitamins, minerals, and amino acids required to regulate insulin and glucose, reproductive hormones, and thyroid function. In women with PCOS, these nutrients can be deficient and may need to be supplemented.

Nutritional Supplement Program for Women with PCOS

- Vitamin D
- Chromium
- N-acetylcysteine (NAC)
- B vitamins
- *D-chiro-inositol* and *pinitol*
- Lecithin
- Antioxidants (selenium, zinc, and vitamins A, C, and E)
- Magnesium

Vitamin D

Vitamin D is sometimes referred to as the "sunshine vitamin." Because our bodies can manufacture this vital nutrient when our skin is exposed to sunshine, vitamin D is not technically a vitamin; we can synthesize vitamin D in our skin. Vitamin D is sometimes classified as a pre-hormone, a hormone being defined as a tissue or glandular secretion released directly into the bloodstream. Like other vitamins, vitamin D can become deficient, and like other hormones, it can become unbalanced.

Following the synthesis of vitamin D in the skin, it is processed in the liver and again in the kidneys to become active. Liver and kidney disease can affect vitamin D status, which can, in turn, contribute to bone disease and exacerbate insulin resistance.

Many readers will be familiar with the importance of vitamin D to the health of our bones and teeth. Because of the growing incidence of osteoporosis (thin bones) and osteopenia (less than optimal density in otherwise normal bones), the medical community has started to increase testing of vitamin D levels. This ramped-up testing is revealing that many of us are low in vitamin D.

Action

Vitamin D supports the absorption, metabolism, and movement of calcium and phosphorus throughout the body. Vitamin D enhances the absorption of calcium from the intestines, its entrance into the bones, and its participation in forming the complex structural scaffolding of mineral in the bones. Intestinal inflammation and disease may also interfere with the absorption of vitamin D. Vitamin D also acts as an immune modulator, helping to combat infections as well as reduce excessive immune responses typical of autoimmune diseases.

Most importantly for women with PCOS, vitamin D supports the action of insulin. Some studies have shown that low levels of vitamin D correlate with insulin resistance.

Supplementation

Supplementation has been shown to relieve some of the symptoms of vitamin D deficiency, and it may improve blood sugar metabolism as well as cellular responses to insulin. There are several forms of vitamin D, notably D2 (ergocalciferol) and D3 (cholecalciferol). Many vitamin D nutritional supplements are in the form of D2, but D3 is thought to be more active and more effective, so it is therefore preferred over D2.

Vitamin D Deficiency

Vitamin D deficiency is known to be associated with insulin resistance, diabetes, and PCOS. Vitamin D is not plentiful in the typical diet, so most vitamin D must come from sunlight or from nutritional supplements. When UV radiation (sunlight) hits our skin, precursor molecules in the skin synthesize vitamin D. One theory on the growing incidence of vitamin D deficiency proposes that we are not exposed to adequate full-spectrum sunlight because we spend more time indoors and shield ourselves from sunlight with sunscreens to prevent skin cancer.

Vitamin D supplementation is often appropriate for women with PCOS and for many others with diabetes, insulin resistance, and metabolic syndrome. The recommended daily allowance (RDA) for vitamin D has changed several times during the past 10 years, but the current RDA is 800 to 2,000 IUs, with some practitioners using significantly higher dosages for selected cases. For women with PCOS, the RDA would be 1,000 to 1,500 IUs as part of a broader treatment protocol.

Vitamin D Deficiency Symptoms

- Muscle pain
- Back and joint pain
- Bone diseases, such as osteoporosis
- Rickets
- Increased susceptibility to colds, flu, infections
- Seasonal affective disorder
- Skin diseases
- Poor wound or burn healing
- Diabetes
- Insulin resistance

Vitamin D Food Sources

Vitamin D is not readily available in the diet, especially in a vegetarian diet. There are no vegetables or fruits that have a high source of vitamin D, although some have minuscule traces. However, D3 can be found in egg yolks, liver, fish oils, and cheese. Cod liver oil and other fish oils have been used medicinally for centuries, and some of the benefits may relate to the D3 content of these oils.

Because of the poor vitamin D content in the diet, many foods are fortified with vitamin D. Milk is commonly enriched with vitamin D, as are many cereals, breads, and some fruit juices. Vitamin D is fat soluble and is best absorbed in the presence of a bit of fat or oil.

Chromium

Chromium is a "trace" mineral, which means that we do not need to consume it in large amounts. Macro minerals, such as calcium and magnesium, are consumed in milligram amounts, while trace minerals are consumed in microgram amounts.

Physicians and nutritionists have used chromium for decades for all manner of blood sugar disorders because chromium enhances the action of insulin. The compound glucose tolerance factor (GTF) is found in the human body and has been shown to play a role in glucose metabolism. Although we don't know much about this compound or the precise structure and actions of GTF, we do know it contains chromium and plays an important role in blood sugar regulation.

Action

Chromium is absorbed from the intestines and is attached to transferrin in order to be transported in the bloodstream. Transferrin is the same molecule that escorts iron around the body. Insulin promotes the transport of chromium into cells, where it becomes bound to a peptide called apochromodulin. Each molecule of apochromodulin can bind with four atoms of chromium, at which point the entire molecular structure is referred to as chromodulin.

One function of chromodulin is to amplify the signal inside the cell following the binding of insulin onto the outside of the cell. Insulin receptors are embedded in cell membranes, and when insulin binds to these receptors, a cascade of events is initiated inside the cell, starting with the activation of intracellular enzymes. Chromodulin has been shown to improve cellular response to insulin. If cells are not responding well to insulin (insulin resistance), chromium can have a therapeutic effect on insulin regulation, which can help women with PCOS. Because brewer's yeast and hibiscus are some of the richest sources of chromium, these agents are emphasized in the recipe and nutrient suggestions of the book.

Chromium also supports serotonin, a neurotransmitter in the brain, and plays a role in the metabolism of cholesterol and nucleic acids, the building blocks of DNA. Chromium acts as an antioxidant and helps to protect the blood vessels from fats.

Chromium Supplementation

There are several forms of chromium: some are industrial and some are nutritional. It is important to know the difference. Trivalent chromium is the only form of chromium that should be supplemented. Hexavalent chromium is more a metal than a nutrient and is not meant to be ingested orally.

Trivalent chromium is available in a variety of molecular forms. It is typically chelated, which means is it bound to a variety of other molecules to create a stable form. These chelated forms are thought to enhance the absorption of chromium, and they include chromium picolinate, chromium aspartate, and chromium polynicotinate. Chromium picolinate is probably the most common and readily available form of chromium nutritional supplement. The RDA for chromium is just 25 micrograms, but most physicians dose chromium at 200 micrograms one or more times a day.

PCOS facts

Chromium Deficiency

Chromium deficiency is associated with poor blood sugar control and with fat deposition in the arteries. In animal studies, severe chromium deficiency has been associated with poor growth and a short lifespan. Our need for chromium increases in times of mental and emotional stress, as well as following physical injuries and traumas. At times of stress, hormonal responses help the body burn more glucose to respond to the stress and more chromium will be needed at these times. Long-term stress can contribute to chromium deficiency, which, in turn, can contribute to insulin resistance and endocrine imbalances, both, in turn, contributing to PCOS.

Caution

Chromium in excess is not associated with any particular toxicity symptoms, but chromium is processed in the liver and kidneys, so individuals with liver or renal disease should avoid supplements in excess of the recommended dosage range. Because chromium enhances insulin response and can cause blood sugar to drop, people taking drugs for diabetes should seek professional guidance before making chromium supplements a part of their supplementation plan.

Chromium may play a role in the prevention or treatment of the following health conditions:

- Acne
- Glaucoma
- High cholesterol levels
- High triglyceride levels
- Hypoglycemia
- Obesity
- Psoriasis
- Type 2 diabetes
- Insulin resistance
- PCOS

Food Sources of Chromium

Chromium is only found in trace amounts in the typical diet. Many whole grains contain chromium in their outer hulls, referred to as the bran, but these grains are often processed, or milled, in such a way that the chromium is lost. Whole grains that have not been milled contain more chromium than those that have been milled. Because much of the grain consumed in the typical U.S. diet is in the form of refined flours, many people consume very little chromium. High-sugar and high-carbohydrate diets also create situations in the kidneys that make it hard to hold on to chromium and other minerals and they are lost in the urine.

Grains also contain phytic acid, a naturally occurring organic acid known to bind to minerals and inhibit their absorption. A high consumption of bread and other processed grains, therefore, is doubly damaging to chromium levels in the body because this kind of diet inhibits the absorption of chromium and impairs the ability of the kidneys to retain it. Antacids, such as calcium carbonate, also may interfere with the absorption of chromium in the digestive tract.

In addition to whole grains, chromium is found in some bran cereals, molasses, eggs, some lean meats, oysters, onions, tomatoes, and brewer's yeast. Hibiscus flowers have the highest known chromium concentration of any naturally occurring plant-based food. Brewer's yeast is added to many of the recipes in this book, and a recipe for high-chromium herbal tea appears on page 144 with the goal of increasing the chromium content of the daily diet.

Q. What is brewer's yeast?

A. Brewer's yeast is a byproduct of brewing alcohol, particularly beer, and is the richest known source of chromium. Brewer's yeast is a specific strain of yeast known as *Saccharomyces cerevisiae* (related to the Spanish word for beer, "cerveza"). Brewer's yeast contains chromium in the form of glucose tolerance factor (GTF). GTF was first identified in 1957 when it was noted to improve glucose control in rats.

For women with PCOS, adding small amounts of brewer's yeast to foods every day will significantly increase chromium in the diet. Two tablespoons (30 mL) of brewer's yeast provides around 120 micrograms of chromium. However, because brewer's yeast has a strong and somewhat bitter flavor, it is difficult to eat in anything more than a teaspoon (5 mL) here and there. Nonetheless, these small amounts consumed regularly can greatly boost your chromium intake and is preferred by some people over purchasing and taking chromium supplements.

So-called nutritional yeast — although highly nutritious — is not the same as brewer's yeast and lacks the chromium content. If in doubt, check the source and verify the nutritional profile. Some of the recipes in this book use brewer's yeast for the purpose of increasing the chromium content of the meal.

Herbs with Traces of Chromium

The following foods and herbs contain small amounts of chromium. Eating these foods regularly can help provide needed chromium, but for chromium deficiency or insulin resistance, more concentrated forms of chromium, such as chromium supplements and brewer's yeast, are needed. The plants named here are listed in descending order, starting with the highest chromium content. Some of these plants will only be familiar to chefs, herbalists, botanists, and gardeners, but all are readily available at herb shops for teas, culinary spices, and — in the case of oats — plain eating.

Herb	Amount of chromium
Hibiscus sabdariffa: hibiscus flowers and calyx	54 mcg/gm
Taraxacum officinale: dandelion leaves	50 mcg/gm
Avena sativa: oats (especially oat bran)	39 mcg/gm
Stevia rebaudiana: sweet leaf	39 mcg/gm
Cymbopogon citratus: lemongrass	37 mcg/gm
Juniperus communis: juniper fruit/berries	32 mcg/gm
Trifolium pratense: red clover	31 mcg/gm
Hordeum vulgare: barley grass (not the grain)	31 mcg/gm
Turnera diffusa: damiana leaf	31 mcg/gm
Elettaria cardamomum: cardamom fruit	30 mcg/gm
Barosma betulina: buchu leaf	29 mcg/gm
Coriandrum sativum: coriander seeds	29 mcg/gm
Nepeta cataria: catnip	27 mcg/gm
Rhodymenia palmata: dulse plant (seaweed)	27 mcg/gm
Dioscorea sp.: wild yam root	26 mcg/gm
Achillea millefolium: yarrow plant	25 mcg/gm
Hydrangea arborescens: hydrangea root	25 mcg/gm
Petasites japonicus: butterbur plant	22 mcg/gm
Equisetum arvense: horsetail plant	22 mcg/gm

N-Acetylcysteine

N-acetylcysteine (NAC) is an amino acid–based compound used to help treat respiratory mucus, cystic fibrosis, chronic bronchitis, and symptoms of respiratory congestion. NAC is sometimes used in an inhalant form. NAC is also showing promise for improving insulin resistance in women with PCOS.

PCOS facts

NAC Research

One clinical study reported in the journal *Fertility and Sterility* was conducted on women with PCOS. The study supplemented women with NAC at a dose of 1.8 to 3 grams per day depending on body weight and reported improved insulin sensitivity after 5 to 6 weeks. Another study published in the same journal reported improved conception rates in women with PCOS-related anovulation when 600 milligrams of NAC per day was used in tandem with a standard fertility drug, clomiphene, when the women had failed to conceive previously with clomiphene therapy alone. The women were given the medications for 5 days starting at day 3 of their menstrual cycles.

NAC has also been shown to improve pregnancy rates with a surgical procedure known as "ovarian drilling." Another small study investigated the combination of NAC with the amino acid arginine in women with PCOS with lack of, or irregular, menstrual cycles and reported improvements in menstrual regularity.

B Vitamins

There is hardly an enzyme system or a chemical reaction in the body that does not involve a B vitamin at least peripherally. For PCOS, many B vitamins play roles in hormonal regulation, fat and sugar metabolism, and basic metabolic and homeostatic functions everywhere in the body. B vitamins are safe and readily available. They should be part of a nutritional supplement routine for women with hormonal imbalances, PCOS, insulin resistance, infertility, and diabetes.

D-chiro-Inositol, Myo-Inositol, and *Pinitol*

D-chiro-inositol and *myo-inositol* are two types of inositol. Inositols are carbohydrate-like molecules, sometimes said to be in the B vitamin family and classified as B vitamin relatives.

Because our own bodies can manufacture various inositols, they are not true vitamins. *D-chiro-inositol* is found in egg yolks, buckwheat (particularly the outer bran), soybeans, and other beans. *Pinitol* is a related substance also found in beans.

Action

D-chiro-inositol and the related *myo-inositol* can both act as "second messengers," agents that enable biochemical signals to be relayed from the cell membrane inward to the nucleus of the cell. In the case of PCOS and insulin resistance, *D-chiro-inositol* and *myo-inositol* promote signals from insulin receptors to the interior of the cell. Both substances occur naturally in the body and play important roles in reproductive function. For example, *myo-inositol* is found in developing egg follicles in human ovaries, and the content of *myo-inositol* is said to be a good indicator of the health and viability of the eggs.

PCOS facts

Symptom Reversal with Inositol Compounds

Several studies have shown that these inositols improve insulin resistance in women with PCOS. Elevated androgens and menstrual irregularities in women with PCOS may respond to *D-chiro-inositol* supplementation. *D-chiro-inositol* is also showing promise for metabolic syndrome because it can help lower triglycerides, cholesterol, and blood pressure. *Myo-inositol* is reported to support the health of eggs in ovarian follicles.

One study, reported in the journal *Gynecological Endocrinology*, showed that 120 women with PCOS who took *myo-inositol* improved the likelihood of achieving pregnancy. In this study, one group was continuously given metformin and the other was given *myo-inositol* with folic acid — a selected few of the group also took follicle-stimulating hormone (FSH). It was shown that 18% of the metformin group achieved pregnancy and 30% of the group receiving *myo-inositol* became pregnant in the initial phase of the study.

Pinitol

In molecular structure, *pinitol* is similar to *D-chiro-inositol*, technically defined as *3-O-methyl-D-chiro-inositol*. *Pinitol* occurs naturally in legumes and citrus and likely contributes to many of the glucose-regulating and insulin-enhancing effects of a diet high in beans. One study dosed a group of type 2 diabetes patients with D-*pinitol* at a dose of 600 milligrams twice a day and reported that improvements in insulin resistance were noted in 3 months.

Food Sources of D-chiro-inositol

Soy lecithin	1,200 mg / 100 g
Carob	1,000 mg / 100 g
Chickpeas	760 mg / 100 g
Brown rice	700 mg / 100 g
Wheat germ	690 mg / 100 g
Lentils	410 mg / 100 g
Barley	390 mg / 100 g
Oats	320 mg / 100 g
Alfalfa	240 mg / 100 g
Beef	260 mg / 100 g
Oranges	210 mg / 100 g
Peanuts	210 mg / 100 g
Molasses	180 mg / 100 g
Peas	160 mg / 100 g
Grapefruits	150 mg / 100 g
Strawberries	95 mg / 100 g
Cauliflower	92 mg / 100 g
Buckwheat bran	85 mg / 100 g

Antioxidants

Thousands of studies have been performed to explore the many health benefits associated with antioxidant nutrients in the diet. And those with chronic inflammatory or degenerative disorders, such as PCOS and diabetes, have a lot to gain from these molecular substances. The main antioxidant nutrients are vitamins A, C, and E, and the minerals zinc and selenium.

Bioflavonoids, plentiful in colorful fruits and vegetables, offer many health benefits as well, including their function as a powerful antioxidant. Aim to eat five or six colorful fruits and vegetables daily — carrots, green leafy veggies, broccoli, and berries. Metabolic syndrome and diabetes both involve inflammatory processes due to elevated sugar and cholesterol in the blood. Bioflavonoids can help protect the blood vessels and tissues from damage. Many bioflavonoids also have positive effects on hormone metabolism that may benefit women with PCOS.

Magnesium

Magnesium is the fourth most abundant mineral in the human body: half of it is found in the bones and the other half is distributed throughout the cells and tissues. Magnesium is required for carbohydrate metabolism, blood sugar regulation, and blood pressure regulation. Low magnesium levels are associated with heart disease, diabetes, high blood pressure, insulin resistance, metabolic syndrome, and PCOS.

PCOS facts

Magnesium Research

One study of more than 200 women, published in the journal *Gynecological Endocrinology*, compared magnesium levels of women with PCOS and women without PCOS. Women with PCOS were shown to be 19 times more likely to have low magnesium levels than women without PCOS. Another study reported that between 25% and 38% of people with type 2 diabetes have low magnesium levels, and that magnesium deficiency correlated with the worst degree of nerve damage and heart disease in people with diabetes. Magnesium supplementation is reported to correlate with improved glucose control and insulin resistance in people with type 2 diabetes. Magnesium can be incorporated into the diet by eating dark green leafy greens, legumes, and whole grains.

Food Sources of Magnesium

- Almonds
- Avocados
- Bananas
- Barley
- Buckwheat
- Cashews
- Cocoa nibs
- Cornmeal
- Flaxseeds
- Green leafy vegetables
- Halibut
- Kelp
- Legumes
- Milk
- Nettles
- Oats
- Peanuts
- Pine nuts
- Poppy seeds
- Pumpkin seeds
- Raisins
- Wheat bran
- Wheat germ
- Yogurt, plain

Q. I have been diagnosed with PCOS. Can I get all the nutrients I need from food sources or do I need to take supplements?

A. There is no definitive answer here. If you like to cook and have the time, motivation, and palate to embrace all of the healthy foods presented in this book, you do not necessarily need to take supplements. However, if you are having serious health challenges, don't like to cook, and are less than enthusiastic about making the required dietary changes, you might benefit greatly from supplements. I start the majority of my patients on supplements, and then spend the next 3 months, if not a year, teaching them about healthy shopping, eating, and cooking until we get them to the point where we can eliminate some, most, or even all of the supplements.

Chapter 5

Herbal Medicines for Managing PCOS

CASE HISTORY

Sarah

When she first came to our clinic, Sarah was a 25-year-old recent college grad taking a bit of time off from school to spend the summer with her parents and save up some money. She was planning on starting a graduate program in the fall. Sarah started her menses at age 14 and had regular cycles for several years, but by the time she was 17, she was having only three or four menses per year, and while in college, they stopped altogether.

Sarah was not obese and had normal blood glucose, cholesterol levels, and thyroid function tests, but she was complaining of increased facial hair and her serum testosterone was slightly elevated. A pelvic ultrasound revealed multiple small cysts on both ovaries.

Treating Sarah for PCOS was challenging. She was very athletic and she was already eating a quality diet. Her healthy lifestyle was preventing the emergence of glucose and cholesterol issues and helped her to maintain an optimal weight. Still, her menstrual cycle was irregular, her fertility was disrupted, and her facial hair remained.

We decided to implement herbal therapy. Sarah was started on an herbal tincture of equal parts *Vitex agnus-castus* (chaste tree), *Serenoa repens* (saw palmetto), and *Glycyrrhiza glabra* (licorice). She called 2 weeks later to say that she had had her first menses in more than 3 years. Sarah continued to take the tincture and she experienced regular monthly cycles. Long-term use of these hormone supportive tinctures appeared to halt the emergence of additional coarse facial and body hair. Sarah's testosterone level also returned to normal levels when checked about a year after starting the herbal tincture.

Several years after her first visit to our clinic, Sarah went on a summer road trip and decided not to bother with the tincture. Her menses stopped immediately. When the trip ended 2 months later, she restarted the tincture treatment and her menses returned.

In addition to specific nutrients that help manage PCOS symptoms and causes, there are several medicinal herbs that are effective in managing PCOS symptoms and causes. These herbs can reduce insulin resistance, lower elevated androgens and prolactin, regulate thyroid, and enhance circulation in the reproductive organs to improve fertility. Any one herb can have an impact on more than one organ or system, and in some cases, a combination of various herbs can be synergistic, becoming even more effective when combined in specific, individualized formulas.

For the most aggressive herbal strategies to treat PCOS, diabetes, or metabolic syndrome, consult a naturopathic physician or licensed herbalist to customize an herbal medicine formula just for you — and to ensure the quality and safety of the products. The herbs we recommend are all safe and nourishing. Nevertheless, before using medicinal herbs, be sure to check with your physician, especially if you are taking any medications.

Herbs to Reduce Insulin Resistance and Control Glucose Levels

Opuntia ficus-indica (Prickly Pear Cactus)

Prickly pear cactus species, including *Opuntia ficus-indica*, is an herb that improves insulin resistance. Prickly pear fruits yield a beautiful magenta flesh and the juice has a delicious flavor, something like a cross between strawberries and watermelon. Opuntia juice can help treat PCOS by controlling blood sugar and improving fat metabolism.

PCOS facts

Opuntia Research

Research studies have shown that opuntia helps to normalize and optimize basic metabolism, including normal blood glucose and cholesterol in animal models of diabetes. Opuntia juice lowered elevated blood sugar in diabetic animals and helped improve glucose control. One clinical trial on patients with metabolic syndrome investigated the efficacy of opuntia on blood fats. Opuntia was found to lower total cholesterol, HDL and LDL, as well as triglycerides, in as few as 14 days. Other studies have confirmed that opuntia can reduce blood fats and promote the liver and muscles to take in glucose, which not only gets the damaging fats and sugars out of the bloodstream, but it assists those tissues in using, or "burning," fats and sugars.

Quick Reference Guide to Medicinal Herbs for PCOS

These herbs address the three chief characteristics of PCOS:

1. Increased insulin resistance
2. Elevated androgen hormones
3. Dysfunctional thyroid

Glucose Management
Herbs to Reduce Insulin Resistance and Control Glucose Levels

- *Opuntia ficus-indica* (prickly pear cactus)
- *Stevia rebaudiana* (stevia)
- *Lepidium meyenii* (maca)
- *Pueraria tuberosa* (pueraria, Indian kudzu)
- *Astragalus membranaceus* (milkvetch)
- *Medicago sativa* (alfalfa)
- *Glycyrrhiza glabra* (licorice)
- *Trigonella foenum-graceum* (fenugreek)
- *Vaccinium* species (blueberries, bilberries)
- *Mahonia aquifolium* (Oregon grape)
- *Hydrastis canadensis* (goldenseal)
- *Silybum marianum* (milk thistle)

Hormone Management
Herbs to Reduce Testosterone, Lower Prolactin, Control Thyroid Hormones, and Regulate Menstrual Cycles

- *Vitex agnus-castus* (chaste tree berry)
- *Glycyrrhiza glabra* (licorice)
- *Serenoa repens* (saw palmetto)
- *Commiphora mukul* (guggul)

Blood Circulation and Lipid Management
Herbs to Enhance Blood Circulation and Manage Blood Lipids

- *Ginkgo biloba* (maidenhair tree)
- *Allium cepa* (onions)
- *Allium sativum* (garlic)
- *Hibiscus sabdariffa* (hibiscus)

Herbs to Increase Omega-3 Essential Fatty Acids

- *Oenothera biennis* (evening primrose)
- *Ribes* species (currant seed)
- *Linum ussitatissimum* (flaxseed)

Stevia rebaudiana (Stevia)

Stevia appears to improve insulin resistance and can be recommended for people with diabetes because it has a glycemic index of zero and has no calories. It is reported to both improve insulin output from the pancreas for type 1 diabetes and improve insulin resistance in type 2 diabetes. Stevia is also naturally high in chromium, making it especially valuable for treating PCOS. Due to its non-caloric, non-glycemic nature, stevia may help to satisfy the sweet tooth for women struggling to avoid soda pop, candy, and other sugary treats.

Recent Stevia Research

One animal study reported that stevia protected the insulin-producing cells in the pancreas from drugs that typically harm them. Stevioside, one of the most studied compounds in stevia, has been credited with reducing blood pressure, blood sugar, and blood fats, while improving both insulin production in the pancreas and insulin sensitivity in cells. Studies have also suggested that stevioside can help lower blood pressure. Whole stevia leaf may reduce the synthesis of glucose in the liver by affecting the enzymes involved in the process, but isolated stevioside lacked this effect.

Lepidium meyenii (Maca)

Maca grows exclusively at high elevations in the Andes, particularly in Peru. Locals often give coca leaves and maca powder to Andes newcomers to combat altitude sickness. Maca belongs to the crucifer family, along with broccoli, cabbage, and Brussels sprouts. This plant family has been shown to have numerous hormonal-balancing and anticancer effects. Maca is nourishing and may help support hormonal and blood sugar balance. It has no known toxicity. Maca powder is now sold around the world for infertility, menopausal symptoms, erectile dysfunction, and cardiovascular disease. The Incas report that maca is a reproductive and circulatory tonic.

Maca contains linoleic and linolenic essential fatty acids and is noted to improve blood fats when included in animal feed. Animal studies have also shown that maca can reduce high blood pressure by enhancing the kidney's ability to process sodium, potassium, and chloride. Maca may also improve blood flow in the heart, which would explain why maca has been used for thousands of years as a treatment for altitude sickness and as a way to improve stamina in low-oxygen situations.

Other researchers investigating maca for metabolic syndrome report that it prevented the development of high cholesterol and blood sugar in rats fed a high-sucrose diet. General hypoglycemic effects have also been reported. One group of researchers reported that maca increased the urinary excretion of glucose, thereby reducing blood levels.

How to Use Maca

Maca can be ground into a fine powder and the flavor is not objectionable. It may be used as a flour substitute in many baked goods. Maca powder may also be stirred into juices, milks, and fruit purées to enhance the medicinal value of the food.

Astragalus membranaceus (Milkvetch)

Astragalus is another legume family herb that has been widely used in herbal medicine for many centuries. Astragalus roots contain saponins that may help protect tissues and reduce inflammation caused by high blood sugar. Astragalus may improve insulin response in cells. Astragalus may also improve high blood sugar by helping the liver and the muscles take up glucose and use it for fuel or convert it to less harmful storage forms. The polysaccharides in *Astragalus membranaceus* are credited with the ability to enhance insulin-signaling pathways in muscle cells, and one small human clinical trial reported reduced insulin resistance in subjects with diabetes. Astragalus also has immune-modulating benefits for chronic infections and allergic conditions. Many traditional Chinese medicines use astragalus in medicinal soups. It has a mild, starchy flavor. Astragalus appears very safe. It is available in herb shops in the form of shredded roots and powders, as well as in tinctures, pills, and formulas. Dried roots are available thinly sliced, and with prolonged simmering in soups yield something edible that resembles bamboo shoots in consistency.

Medicago sativa (Alfalfa)

Alfalfa is another legume family herb that contains saponins as well as *D-chiro-inositol*. Alfalfa has been a traditional folkloric herbal remedy for diabetes, and modern research has suggested alfalfa might enhance glucose metabolism. Alfalfa in the form of alfalfa sprouts may benefit hormonal regulation by delivering phytoestrogens, and phytoestrogens are credited with preventing heart disease, cancer, and menopausal symptoms. Alfalfa leaf teas and products are non-toxic, extremely nourishing, and support healthy hormonal regulation. Alfalfa seeds for making your own sprouts are also widely available and can be sprouted at home.

Glycyrrhiza glabra (Licorice)

Licorice is another legume family member that has many hormonal and metabolic regulatory properties. Something as simple and inexpensive as drinking licorice tea can be a part of an overall treatment approach for PCOS. A saponin in glycyrrhiza named glycyrrhizic acid is credited with an ability to improve insulin resistance and fat metabolism in animal models of metabolic syndrome. Glycyrrhiza has been found to reduce inflammation and support function in animal models of diabetic kidney damage, improve insulin sensitivity, reduce fat deposition in tissues, and suppress the accumulation in abdominal fat.

Licorice and High Blood Pressure

There have been widely publicized reports that licorice may lead to an increase in blood pressure, though the actual occurrence of this side effect is quite rare. Nevertheless, high blood pressure is a concern for some women with metabolic syndrome. Studies are now indicating that licorice may aggravate high blood pressure more often in those with a preexisting complex adrenal disorder involving altered potassium levels. Licorice, in fact, has been reported to reduce blood pressure in animal models of metabolic syndrome. The side effect of elevated blood pressure remains unpredictable, so people using licorice supplements should regularly monitor their blood pressure. People with abnormally low potassium levels should avoid licorice due to the possibility of serious muscle weakness and high blood pressure. Do not consume more than 2 or 3 cups (500 to 750 mL) of licorice tea per day unless under a physician's guidance.

Trigonella foenum-graceum (Fenugreek)

Fenugreek is yet another legume family plant, but rather than producing edible beans, it produces aromatic seeds. Fenugreek seeds have been reported in folkloric literature to be useful for type 2 diabetes. There is limited modern research, but the few studies we do have support the traditional use of this plant. Fenugreek seeds are commonly ground into a spice that has a slightly pungent aromatic quality and a slightly bittersweet flavor that many people liken to maple syrup. Fenugreek seeds may also be sprouted and used as a delicate vegetable in salads and garnishes.

Recent Fenugreek Research

One study reported that fenugreek lowered blood glucose in type 1 diabetic animals "almost" equally to insulin itself, and another study in type 2 diabetic animals showed that fenugreek lowered blood glucose equally to metformin. Fenugreek also improves glucose tolerance and reduces elevated blood fats. Another clinical study investigated the effects of fenugreek

How to Sprout Fenugreek Seeds

Sprouted fenugreek seeds can be eaten whole in salads, or the sprouts can be dried and ground to be used as a flour substitute or mixing component.

1. Place 1 tablespoon (15 mL) of the seeds in a wide-mouthed glass canning jar and cover with 2 cups (500 mL) of water. Let stand 24 hours. You may purchase or make a fine-mesh screen that fits inside the ring of the canning jar, fashion a cheese cloth strainer, or simply leave the jar without a lid and open and drain several times a day through a stainless steel fine-mesh kitchen strainer. Rinse after 24 hours and drain out all the water.

2. After the initial soaking, rinse the seeds thoroughly at least three times a day with fresh tap water, and drain. Store in a dark cool cupboard between rinsings.

3. When the seeds begin to sprout, place the jar in a sunny window and wait for the first tiny leaves to turn green. The fenugreek sprouts are ready to eat immediately or may be dried and ground into flour.

4. To dry sprouts, place on a baking sheet in an oven set to 200°F (100°C) — or use a commercial food dehydrator on Low — until dry. As most ovens do not have a setting as low as needed, it may be necessary to leave the oven door ajar.

on blood sugar in diabetic patients who were not responding well to sulfonylurea drugs. Half of the participants were given fenugreek and the other half a placebo for 12 weeks. The group given the fenugreek pills showed improved fasting blood sugar levels, better glucose control after eating, and better glycosylated hemoglobin.

Like maca powder and bean flours or purées, powdered fenugreek might also be used as a flour substitute in baked goods. One innovative study used fenugreek powder liberally in a bread recipe and reported the bread reduced insulin resistance over 4 hours immediately following consumption compared to an identical-appearing and -tasting "control" wheat bread. The somewhat pungent and slightly bitter flavor of fenugreek limits its use in baking. It might be easiest to add fenugreek powder to various recipes by the teaspoon (5 mL) or tablespoon (15 mL) on a daily basis for a cumulative effect.

Legume Herbal Formula

You can make tea from alfalfa, astragalus, pueraria, fenugreek, or licorice. You can also blend these herbs. This formula will fill a sandwich-sized sealable plastic bag. Store the tea in a dark cool place.

Legume Herbal Tea

2 oz	alfalfa leaves, dried	60 g
2 oz	astragalus root, shredded	60 g
1 oz	licorice root, shredded	30 g

1. Blend the dried ingredients.
2. In a tea kettle, bring water to a full boil.
3. Place 1 tbsp (15 mL) of the dried herb mixture per cup (250 mL) of water in a teapot or saucepan.
4. Steep the herbal tea mixture for 10 minutes.
5. Strain. Use a wire mesh strainer, muslin bag, or special tea pot with built-in ceramic or mesh strainer. You can prepare a single cup using a tea ball or small 1-cup (250 mL) strainer or prepare an entire potful. To prepare larger batches, put the herbs loose in a pan, cover with boiling water for 10 minutes and strain. You may also use a French press, throwing the herbs in the bottom instead of coffee.
6. Aim to drink 3 or more cups (750 mL) per day for best medicinal effects.

Vaccinium species
Blueberries and Bilberries

Blueberry and bilberry leaves and fruit have long been a folk remedy for diabetes. Animal studies have shown that compounds in blueberries can reduce blood glucose and enhance insulin sensitivity in type 2 diabetic mice. One of these mechanisms involves the promotion of the intracellular "second messenger" cyclic adenosine monophosphate (AMP) and the associated protein kinases. Blueberries freeze very well, so purchase them in quantity in the summer to last you all year. Blueberries also make fantastic herbal vinegars, dressings, and sauces.

Recent *Vaccinium* Research

Human studies on glucose regulation are sparse, but one study in overweight and obese women with metabolic syndrome reported that the consumption of blueberries had a slight but statistically significant effect on total weight and waist circumference compared to other berries and isolated chemical concentrates from berries. More widely studied and reported is the ability of flavonoids in vaccinium to have positive and protective effects on blood vessels.

Anthocyanins

All of the *Vaccinium* species are thought to be among the richest sources of anthocyanins. Anthocyanins (also called anthocyanosides) are a group of bluish-purple-pigmented flavonoids found in *Vaccinium* species that have a protective effect on capillaries and blood vessel walls. Anthocyanins are powerful antioxidants and reduce the inflammatory damage to blood vessels inflicted by the many inflammatory and abnormal metabolic processes seen with diabetes, high cholesterol, and metabolic syndrome. Many commercial products are standardized to deliver 160 milligrams of anthocyanins per day. Eating whole blueberries can also be recommended for people with diabetes and those with metabolic syndrome. Many wild species of blueberries exist in Europe and North America, many of which have been traditionally used by indigenous people for the symptoms of diabetes.

Many of the antioxidant and anti-inflammatory effects credited to anthocyanins may be due to a balancing of the genes involved with inflammatory and anti-inflammatory responses (by way of their effects on protein kinase enzymes). These protective effects on blood vessel cells (endothelium) are well documented and appear to extend to the retina and circulation in the eye. Blueberries can be recommended to help protect the vision of people with diabetes.

Anthocyanins may also reduce blood pressure and excessive platelet clumping, thereby reducing the risks of blood clots and cardiovascular disease, for which women with PCOS and metabolic syndrome are at increased risk. Animal studies suggest that *Vaccinium* reduces fat deposits in blood vessels and tightens the connective tissue structure of blood vessels, limiting the ability of fats and cholesterol in the blood to do damage. Anthocyanins, like other flavonoids, promote collagen to "cross-link." Collagen is a component of connective tissue that helps provide strength and structural integrity to tissues, and cross-linking collagen fibers is part of what lends such strength and

> **PCOS facts**
>
> **Blueberries**
>
> Blueberries are believed to enhance circulation and to be preventive and therapeutic for diabetic eye disease and for numbness and tingling due to nerve damage and poor circulation.

flexibility to these fibers. When the connective tissue scaffolding in various tissues and organs is strong, the tissues and organs are less easily damaged by inflammatory processes.

Although not in the *Vaccinium* genus, grapes, cherries, currants, and pomegranates also contain anthocyanins and are credited with cardiovascular protective effects. Hibiscus flowers are another ready dietary source of anthocyanins.

Cranberries

Cranberries are also in the *Vaccinium* species, and investigations suggest that cranberries may also have positive effects on fat and glucose metabolism in metabolic syndrome. One small human study involving the consumption of cranberries reported a significant reduction in cholesterol compared to placebo.

PCOS facts

Red and Purple Pigment Benefits

Many fruits and vegetables that are a bright red, purple, or blue in color, such as blueberries, are high in anthocyanins and prooligomeric cyaninins, the molecular terms for these brightly colored compounds. Most berries contain these healthful compounds and are reported to be powerful antioxidants and to help protect the blood vessels from the damaging effects of high fat and sugar in the bloodstream. Grapes, pomegranates, cherries, blueberries, blackberries, raspberries, and cranberries are good sources of anthocyaninins. Aim to eat as many of these as possible. Try making homemade salad dressing from puréed raspberries, throwing blueberries into a blender for a smoothie drink, adding cherries or cranberries to a vegetable roast, or garnish poached fish with cherries or cranberries. The health benefits of berries and anthocyaninins do not apply to sugar- or fructose-sweetened fruit juices, or to berry-flavored processed foods such as cherry popsicles, Pop-Tarts, or anything other than the whole fruits.

Mahonia aquifolium and *Hydrastis canadensis* (Oregon Grape and Goldenseal)

These herbs promote the liver's metabolism of cholesterol. *Mahonia aquifolium* (formerly *Berberis vulgaris*) goes by the common name Oregon grape, and hydrastis is the fairly well-known goldenseal plant. Both of these bitter roots have been used traditionally to improve digestive and liver function, and both are useful in diabetes and high cholesterol by helping the body to process fats and sugars. These herbs may be included in the treatment of PCOS because they also have a beneficial effect on processing hormones in the body. Because the liver is responsible for metabolizing hormones and excreting them from the body, supporting liver function often improves high-estrogen symptoms, such as breast cysts, bleeding abnormalities, endometriosis, and ovarian cysts.

Both Oregon grape and goldenseal contain the isoquinoline alkaloid berberine. Investigations have shown that berberine can improve insulin resistance in humans. Human clinical trials with people with insulin-resistant diabetes have shown significant reductions in blood glucose, fats, and insulin as evidence of improved insulin response and general metabolism. Researchers in China report that berberine lowers blood fats through numerous complex effects on cellular enzymes, through insulin signals inside cells, and through other direct effects on fat cells.

Silybum marianum (Milk Thistle)

Milk thistle seeds have been noted to support liver function and reduce hyperlipidemia. One placebo-controlled double-blinded trial used 420 milligrams of silymarin, a component of silybum, for a duration of 3 months. Total cholesterol and HDL (good cholesterol) levels were noted to be slightly reduced in those receiving milk thistle compared to the group receiving the placebo. Although the lipid-lowering effects may not be dramatic, the ability of silybum to protect the liver from degeneration due to fat deposits or to exposure to a variety of liver-toxic drugs and chemicals is noteworthy. Any and all people found to have fatty liver or elevated liver enzymes should consider long-term supplementation with silybum. The use of silybum may also enhance fertility and regulate metabolic and

How to Use Milk Thistle

The seeds, which are somewhat similar in size to shelled sunflower seeds, are the part of the plant used as a medicine. Silybum seeds are commonly ground into powders or concentrates and then encapsulated or tinctured. They are available alone or in combination with other products. Silybum seeds may also be purchased in bulk and can be ground in a coffee or other small grinder. Grind them in small batches and work the powder into cooked foods, or combine them with toasted and raw sesame seeds and nut meal, culinary spices, and a bit of salt to use as a sodium substitute on foods.

hormonal imbalances. Many herbalists and physicians use liver herbs as one component of broader therapeutic plans in the treatment of PCOS, ovarian cysts, breast pain and cysts, and PMS. Women with high cholesterol, insulin resistance, digestive disturbances, and hormonal imbalances (PMS and PCOS), or those with a history of using many hormonal pharmaceutical prescriptions, may benefit from taking milk thistle. For anyone with elevated liver enzymes or a history of hepatitis or gallbladder disease, this is doubly true.

Milk Thistle Seedy Salt

While milk thistle pills and tinctures are somewhat expensive, milk thistle seeds are not. They are not tasty enough to eat all on their own, but they are enjoyable when ground and mixed with salt. Use this salt to provide your body with a little liver support everyday while getting some valuable essential fatty acids at the same time. Sprinkle on soups, salads, eggs, and popcorn. Make it fresh every few days.

2 tbsp	milk thistle seeds	30 mL
2 tbsp	sesame seeds	30 mL
1 tbsp	raw walnut pieces	15 mL
1 tbsp	salt	15 mL
1 tbsp	herb or herbs of choice, such as 1 tsp (5 mL) each of cumin seeds, smoked paprika, and dried basil (optional)	15 mL

1. Toast the sesame seeds in a dry skillet. Break the walnuts into small pieces by hand to make grinding easier.

2. Put the sesame and milk thistle seeds, along with walnut pieces, in a coffee grinder reserved for this purpose, or in a seed grinder or nut mill, and grind into a fine to slightly coarse powder as desired. Transfer to a small mixing bowl and combine with the salt, or herbs if desired. Mix well.

3. Transfer to a small jar or shaker.

Herbs to Reduce Testosterone, Lower Prolactin, Control Thyroid Hormones, and Regulate Menstrual Cycles

Vitex agnus-castus (Chaste Tree Berry)

Chaste tree berry has been used for centuries to treat menstrual and fertility disorders in women and is a valuable medicine to consider in a broad treatment protocol for PCOS. Vitex has been shown to increase progesterone levels and to reduce elevated prolactin and testosterone.

PCOS facts

Normalized Testosterone

Animal studies have shown chaste tree to normalize elevated testosterone levels. Many women with PCOS have high testosterone levels, which contribute to the excess facial and body hair and amenorrhea. Chaste tree appears to lower excess testosterone using mechanisms involving neurotransmitters in the brain and their effects on the hypothalamic and pituitary hormones. Specifically, the neurotransmitter dopamine is involved in the regulation of pituitary hormones, which in turn regulate reproductive hormones, including testosterone. Chaste tree has also been shown to bind opiate receptors, which in turn promote dopamine activity.

One clinical trial conducted at Stanford University compared chaste tree and other supportive nutrients to a placebo in 93 women with infertility. After 3 months, progesterone levels in the women on the *Vitex agnus-castus* were increased compared to those women on the placebo medication. What's more, 13 of the 53 women on the *Vitex* achieved pregnancy, while none of the women on the placebo became pregnant.

Because the flavor of chaste tree is not as agreeable as some of the legume herbs, it is prepared less often as an herbal tea. Tinctures and capsules are readily available from physicians and some herbal product vendors. *Vitex agnus-castus* is a common ingredient in commercial herbal formulas to address PMS and menopausal complaints. It can be effective for treating amenorrhea, as well as irregular menses and breast pain.

Glycyrrhiza glabra (Licorice)

In traditional Chinese medicine, licorice has been referred to as "the great harmonizer" due to the belief that it can go everywhere in the body and pull together the actions of other herbs in botanical formulas. Licorice seems to deserve this reputation because it can be used for ulcers, viral infections, fatigue, adrenal disorders, infertility, and numerous hormonal and metabolic regulatory issues. Something as simple and inexpensive as drinking licorice tea can be a part of an overall treatment approach for PCOS.

Glycyrrhizic acid, a saponin in *Glycyrrhiza glabra*, is credited with an ability to improve insulin resistance and fat metabolism in animal models of metabolic syndrome. Licorice has also been found to reduce inflammation and support function in animal models of diabetic kidney damage, improve insulin sensitivity, reduce fat deposition in tissues, and suppress the accumulation of abdominal fat.

Animal studies suggest that licorice can reduce elevated androgens, and one human study has shown that licorice can decrease serum testosterone in women. Licorice is a traditional Japanese herbal medicine used to treat infertility. Several studies have shown that licorice can promote ovulation and menstruation in amenorrheic women, as well as in women with PCOS.

In Japan, to treat PCOS, licorice is often combined with peony in a traditional herbal medicine called shakuyaku-kanzo-to, which is reported to reduce elevated testosterone. Researchers report that licorice helps normalize elevated testosterone by a number of mechanisms, including reducing the synthesis of testosterone and by blocking the dehydrogenase enzymes that help synthesize it.

Licorice may also reduce elevated prolactin. An undesirable side effect of some drugs is prolactin elevation and the cessation of menses. Licorice combinations have been shown to lower prolactin and restore normal menstruation in women using such drugs.

Serenoa repens (Saw Palmetto)

Saw palmetto has been studied for its ability to treat diseases of the prostate, but very little research has been done on its effects with PCOS. Many older herbal books report that saw palmetto is a genitourinary tonic in both sexes. *Serenoa repens* has been shown to reduce the uptake of androgens, including dihydrotestosterone and testosterone, into tissues by 40%. Serenoa berries contain fatty acids known collectively as liposterols and named individually as lauric, oleic, myristic, and linoleic acids. All of these fatty acids have been shown to inhibit the 5-alpha-reductase enzyme. The enzyme 5-alpha-reductase is found in the adrenal glands (and in the prostate) and it converts testosterone into its most active form, dihydrotestosterone. Women with hirsutism and elevated testosterone may have excessive 5-alpha-reductase enzyme activity. *Serenoa repens* may also reduce elevated prolactin by blocking cellular signaling at prolactin receptors.

Commiphora mukul (Guggul)

Guggul has beneficial actions on the thyroid. The steroidal compounds in *Commiphora mukul*, the guggulsterones, are credited with lowering elevated blood fats and sugars through several different mechanisms — by improving metabolism of fat in the liver, by enhancing the uptake of iodine by the thyroid, and by increasing production of thyroid hormones.

Animal studies have also shown that guggulsterones inhibit the development and maturation of fat-storing cells, called adipocytes. Guggulsterones exert a direct inhibitory effect on adipocytes, decreasing the synthesis of new cells, decreasing the fat accumulation in existing cells, and increasing the destruction (apoptosis) of fat cells. Specific proteins associated with adipocyte functions are suppressed by guggul.

Herbs to Enhance Blood Circulation and Manage Blood Lipids

Ginkgo biloba (Maidenhair Tree)

Extensive modern research has been conducted on *Ginkgo biloba* and its effectiveness in treating heart and circulatory diseases. Ginkgo also may be a useful herb for women with PCOS and circulatory concerns, such as elevated glucose, lipids, and blood pressure. Studies show that ginkgo is helpful for supporting circulation to the brain, the extremities, microcirculatory blood vessels, and the heart muscle. Ginkgo can be recommended to treat impaired circulation in people with diabetes, and to decrease the risk of ischemic stroke (stroke caused by an interruption in the flow of blood to the brain), clot formation, and heart disease in women with PCOS and metabolic syndrome. Animal studies suggest that ginkgo can help prevent the accumulation of advanced glycation end products in diabetic rats. Gingko supplements are especially important for older women with PCOS and high blood pressure.

Allium cepa (Onions) and *Allium sativum* (Garlic)

Onions and garlic are two Liliaceae family bulbs that may support healthy blood glucose, cholesterol, and blood pressure. Several sulfur-containing constituents — allyl propyl disulfide (APDS) and diallyl disulfide oxide (allicin) — are believed to contribute to many of the medicinal effects.

How to Use Onions and Garlic

Garlic is more extensively studied and may be more powerful than onions, but both garlic and onions should be used extensively and liberally in the diet for their numerous health benefits. Those who do not tolerate raw onions or garlic due to digestive side effects are often able to tolerate baked, boiled, or otherwise cooked onions and garlic. Aim to keep fresh garlic and onions around as a kitchen staple and work them into every possible vegetable, meat, egg, and other dish. Onions can even be puréed in a blender to create a liquid base for soups and sauces.

Garlic was shown to reduce blood glucose, improve insulin sensitivity, and reduce oxidative stress in animal models of diabetes fed a high-fructose diet. Animal studies also suggest that garlic may help protect the heart from the damage that occurs in diabetes. Garlic inhibits the clumping of platelets, which can occur excessively in diabetes and metabolic syndrome due to inflammation in the blood, and which can contribute to the increased risk for clots seen in these conditions.

How to Eat More Garlic

Sometimes it is tempting not to bother with the garlic when you have to stop and break apart the bulbs and peel all the cloves. If you have the cloves ready to use, you are more likely to eat more.

1. Keep one of the commercial minced garlic products on hand. Small 2-ounce (30 g) jars are available in most modern grocery stores.

2. Try spending a half an hour now and then peeling 4 or 5 or more whole bulbs of garlic and removing the papery covering from the individual cloves. These peeled cloves will store for several months, covered with olive oil in a glass jar in the refrigerator. Either spoon out individual cloves as needed, or use a spoonful of the cloves along with some of the oil in cooking.

3. Make small batches of garlic oil purée to use in dressings, sauces, and cooking. Put peeled cloves in the blender with either olive or quality nut oils and purée. Put the whole purée in a small jar and store in the refrigerator to spoon into whatever you are cooking.

4. Make garlic vinegar. Prepare as the above garlic oil but purée with vinegar of choice (apple cider, balsamic, wine, etc.) instead of oil, and store the vinegar/garlic purée in a small canning jar. You may leave the garlic in and consume along with the vinegar. Or you can shake the jar every day for several weeks and strain the garlic particulate out through muslin or a cheesecloth-lined wire mesh strainer to yield a clear liquid. Vinegars have a long shelf life and can be used in sauces, stir-fries, salad dressings, and vegetable dishes.

Hibiscus sabdariffa (Hibiscus)

Species of hibiscus are beautiful flowering shrubs found in tropical regions. Their flowers can be used to make a sour-tasting tea that has numerous medicinal benefits. The bright red, pink, orange, and other anthocyanin pigments in hibiscus may help protect the blood vessels from the damaging effects of high blood glucose and high blood pressure, and animal studies suggest that the anthocyanins reduce the ability of LDL cholesterol to form atherosclerotic lesions inside blood vessels. Hibiscus also helps protect the tissue from the inflaming effects of advanced glycation end products, and it is also very high in chromium, which may contribute to its blood sugar–balancing effects in PCOS.

High-Chromium Hibiscus

According to the USDA phytochemical database, hibiscus flowers are the highest plant source of chromium, containing 54 micrograms of chromium per gram of dried flowers. Drinking hibiscus flower tea sweetened with dried stevia leaves, which also contain chromium, may meet your nutritional need for chromium in treating PCOS. A single cup (250 mL) of tea can contain 100 micrograms of chromium, making it possible to get your 200 micrograms per day with a just a couple of cups of tea. Hibiscus and stevia combine well with licorice, alfalfa, and other herbs noted to improve hormonal balance.

Recent Hibiscus Research

One human clinical trial involving 60 people with diabetes evaluated the effects of *Hibiscus sabdariffa* tea on blood lipids. Patients were randomly divided into two groups and given either black tea or hibiscus tea, which they drank twice daily for a month. The patients receiving the hibiscus tea showed significantly lower lipids compared to the group receiving the black tea.

High-Chromium Herbal Tea

3 oz	hibiscus flowers	90 g
2 oz	stevia leaves	60 g
2 oz	alfalfa leaves	60 g
1 oz	fenugreek seeds, freshly ground	30 g

1. Combine the hibiscus flowers, stevia leaves, alfalfa leaves, and fenugreek seeds in a small sealable bag or glass jar.
2. Steep one heaping tablespoon (15 mL) per cup (250 mL) of hot water. Aim to drink 3 or more cups (750 mL or more) each day.

Herbs to Increase Omega-3 Essential Fatty Acids

Oils from the herbs *Oenothera biennis* (evening primrose), *Ribes* species (currant seed), and *Linum usitatissimum* (flaxseed) help normalize cholesterol and reduce inflammation. These essential fatty acids (EFAs) have numerous anti-inflammatory benefits for people with diabetes and metabolic syndrome.

EFAs are very sensitive to heat and light. Flax, currant, and other seed oils can go rancid more quickly than other fixed oils. For this reason, care should be taken to buy the freshest oils available, store them airtight in the refrigerator, and use them up quickly. Because they are heat sensitive, it is better to use the more stable olive, coconut, and walnut oils in baking or frying, and use the delicate seed oils in sauces, dressings, and blender drinks.

Part 3

Recipes

Meal Plans

This four-week meal plan will help you follow a PCOS dietary program using the recipes in this book, along with other common foods. To maximize the benefit of this meal plan, use the nutrient boosts included with each day, as well as the PCOS boosts outlined with the recipes (when applicable). Add 1 tbsp (15 mL)

❧ Week 1

	Monday	Tuesday	Wednesday
Breakfast	Blueberry Smoothie* Hard-cooked egg Celery sticks and cucumber slices Hibiscus Herb Tea*	Piquant White Bean and Parsley Dip* Pico de Gallo* Bell pepper and zucchini slices 2 high-fiber whole-grain crackers Medicinal Mint Tea*	Lentil-Stuffed Tomatoes* Astragalus Tea*
Snack	2 apple slices spread with 2 tsp (10 mL) almond butter Prickly Pear Power Punch*	Piña Macolada*	½ cup (125 mL) soy nuts ½ banana Prickly Pear Power Punch*
Lunch	Snow Pea and Bell Pepper Salad* 2 high-fiber whole-grain crackers ½ oz (15 g) sliced cheese	Marinated Vegetable Salad* 2 high-fiber whole-grain crackers Italian White Bean Spread*	Carrot and Ginger Soup* Yogurt Dill Dip with Belgian Endive* Fresh fruit slices
Snack	½ pear ¼ cup (60 mL) raw pecans Winter Tea*	Pomegranate Apricot Fizz* Carrot sticks	Prickly Pear Spritzer* ½ cup (125 mL) raw almonds
Dinner	Caramelized Onion and Roasted Mushroom Soup* Poached Fish Jardinière* Steamed asparagus	Grilled Chicken with Stir-Fried Vegetables* Personal Garden Herb Salad*	Carrot Ginger Soup* Oriental Fish Fillets* Cooked greens (mustard, kale or collard greens)
Nutrient Boosts	Sprinkle 1 to 2 tsp (5 to 10 mL) nutritional yeast on soup	Add ¼ tsp (1 mL) brewer's yeast to bean dip and to Pico de Gallo Sprinkle 1 tsp (5 mL) sesame seeds on salad	Drizzle 1 tsp (5 mL) flaxseed oil on cooked greens

* The recipe is in the book; unless otherwise indicated, the amount is one serving.

inositol powder to each serving of herbal tea or other beverage if it is not already included in the recipe. Supplement with vitamin D, N-acetylcysteine, magnesium, chromium picolinate, and a combination antioxidant containing selenium and vitamins A, C, and E, as recommended by your health practitioner.

Thursday	Friday	Saturday	Sunday
Oven-Roasted Asparagus* Hard-cooked egg Melon slice Cinnamon Tea*	1 oz (30 g) canned herring or sardines Hard-cooked egg ½ banana Elderberry Tea*	Raspberry Yogurt Smoothie* 1 apricot, plum or peach Flor de Jamaica Tea*	Kitchen Sink Frittata* Melon slice Summer Tea*
Prickly Pear Power Punch*	4 to 5 figs 4 to 5 raw Brazil nuts Prickly Pear Power Punch*	½ oz (15 g) canned herring 2 high-fiber whole-grain crackers Prickly Pear Power Punch*	½ nectarine ¼ cup (60 mL) raw cashews Prickly Pear Power Punch*
Grilled Stuffed Jalapeño Peppers* 1 cup (250 mL) grapes ½ cup (125 mL) low-fat cottage cheese	Bulgur and Vegetable Lettuce Wraps* 1 cup (250 mL) grapes	Legume Guacamole* Black Bean Salsa* Carrot sticks and red bell pepper slices	Mango Chicken Wrap* Jicama slices
Jalapeño Punch* Melon slice	Almond Milk* 1 cup (250 mL) grapes or cherries	Rose Essence Nectar* ½ nectarine	Hard-cooked egg Baby carrots
Thai-Style Squash Soup* Stir-Fried Vegetables with Tofu*	Vegetarian Chili* Spinach and Grapefruit Salad* Steamed broccoli	Tandoori Haddock* Chickpea Curry* Braised Brussels sprouts	Curried Butternut Squash and Bean Soup* Broiled salmon Cooked kale
Sprinkle ½ to 1 tsp (2 to 5 mL) nutritional yeast on cottage cheese and on stir-fry	Sprinkle ½ tsp (2 mL) ground flax seeds on chili Drizzle 1 tsp (5 mL) flaxseed oil on broccoli	Sprinkle 1 tsp (5 mL) sesame seeds on guacamole and on salsa Drizzle 1 tsp (5 mL) flaxseed oil on Brussels sprouts	Sprinkle 1 tbsp (15 mL) raw nuts on salmon and kale Drizzle 1 tbsp (15 mL) flaxseed oil or other high-quality oil on kale

❧ *Week 2*

	Monday	Tuesday	Wednesday
Breakfast	Almond Butter Smoothie* Hibiscus Herb Tea*	1 slice whole-grain bread spread with Lemon Pesto* and topped with shredded carrots and canned herring or sardines (or leftover fish from Monday) Medicinal Mint Tea*	Spinach Feta Muffin* Hard-cooked egg ½ grapefruit Astragalus tea*
Snack	½ apple ¼ cup (60 mL) sunflower seeds Prickly Pear Power Punch*	Banana Walnut Smoothie*	Celery stalk spread with almond butter and sprinkled with raisins Prickly Pear Power Punch*
Lunch	Chicken and Bean Salad*	Garden Patch Spinach Salad* Hard-cooked egg	Black-Eyed Pea Salad with Cajun Chicken* Melon slice
Snack	3 dried apricots ¼ cup (60 mL) pecans Prickly Pear Power Punch*	½ pear 4 to 5 raw Brazil nuts Prickly Pear Power Punch*	Cucumber Slushie* Carrot sticks Prickly Pear Power Punch*
Dinner	Poached Fish Jardinière* Ginger Carrots* Roasted Beet, Walnut and Arugula Salad*	Roasted Cauliflower and Red Pepper Soup* Garden Path Burger* Roasted Beet, Walnut and Arugula Salad*	Cilantro Bean Soup* Pepper-Crusted Rainbow Trout* Citrus Fennel Slaw*
Nutrient Boosts	Sprinkle 1 tbsp (15 mL) raw nuts on lunch salad Sprinkle 1 tbsp (15 mL) each raw nuts and flaxseed oil on fish and beets	Drizzle lunch salad with 1 to 2 tsp (5 to 10 mL) flaxseed or other high-quality oil	Sprinkle 1 tbsp (15 mL) raw nuts and 2 tsp (10 mL) flaxseed oil on lunch salad Sprinkle raw walnuts on slaw

* The recipe is in the book; unless otherwise indicated, the amount is one serving.

Thursday	Friday	Saturday	Sunday
Poached egg Leftover soup or salmon from Wednesday Cinnamon Tea*	Scalloped Soybeans* Melon slices Leftover vegetables Elderberry Tea*	Hard-cooked egg Spicy Hummus* Cucumber slices Raw broccoli and cauliflower florets Flor de Jamaica Tea*	Crustless Zucchini Quiche* Summer Tea*
1 cup (250 mL) grapes Prickly Pear Power Punch*	1/2 cup (125 mL) soy nuts Baby carrots Prickly Pear Power Punch*	1/4 cup (60 mL) each soy nuts, raw cashews and dried currants Prickly Pear Power Punch*	1 cooked beet, sliced and drizzled with lemon juice and flax seed oil 1 tbsp (15 mL) raw walnuts Prickly Pear Power Punch*
Marinated Vegetable Salad* Hard-cooked egg 1/2 orange	Veggie Sandwich* 1 cup (250 mL) grapes	Bulgur Salad with Broccoli, Radishes and Celery* Watermelon slice	Piquant Marinated Vegetables* Roasted Red Pepper and Feta Hummus* Cucumber slices 1 cup (250 mL) berries
Agua de Manzana (Apple Water)* Spinach Feta Muffin*	Warm Almond Nutmeg Milk* 1/2 pear	1/2 apple, sliced and spread with 2 tsp (10 mL) almond butter Prickly Pear Power Punch*	Leftover hummus Baby carrots Prickly Pear Power Punch*
Tandoori Haddock* Stir-Fried Chinese Greens* Steamed Asian Vegetable Medley*	Asian Salmon* Citrus Fennel Slaw* Steamed broccoli, kale or collard greens	Ginger Soy Mushroom Soup* Grilled Chicken with Stir-Fried Vegetables* Steamed broccoli, kale, collard greens or mustard greens	Chickpea Hot Pot* Spinach Fancy* Leftover marinated vegetables Melon slices
Sprinkle 1 tbsp (15 mL) raw nuts and 2 tsp (10 mL) flaxseed oil on salad Sprinkle 2 tsp (10 mL) each sesame seeds and flaxseed oil on greens	Sprinkle 1 tbsp (15 mL) raw nuts and 2 tsp (10 mL) flaxseed oil on fish and slaw Sprinkle broccoli with 1 tsp (5 mL) nutritional yeast	Sprinkle 2 tsp (10 mL) flaxseed oil on salad Sprinkle broccoli with 2 tsp (10 mL) nutritional yeast	Top beets with 1 tsp (5 mL) low-fat sour cream

❧ Week 3

	Monday	Tuesday	Wednesday
Breakfast	Maca Mango Smoothie* Hibiscus Herb Tea*	Hard-cooked egg or 1 oz (30 g) canned herring Quick Roasted Red Pepper Dip* Raw cucumber, broccoli and cauliflower pieces Medicinal Mint Tea*	1 oz (30 g) canned herring ½ cup (125 mL) low-fat cottage cheese Melon slice Astragalus Tea*
Snack	4 figs ½ cup (125 mL) raw pecans Prickly Pear Power Punch*	Coffee Carob Smoothie*	Carrot sticks ¼ cup (60 mL) raw cashews Prickly Pear Power Punch*
Lunch	Black-Eyed Pea Salad with Cajun Chicken* 1 nectarine	Carrot and Ginger Soup* Colorful Bean and Corn Salad*	Grilled Stuffed Jalapeño Peppers* 1 oz (30 g) canned herring 1 cup (250 mL) grapes
Snack	Carrot sticks Prickly Pear Power Punch*	Blueberry Prickly Pear Spritzer* Cucumber slices	Watermelon Slushie* Pumpkin Millet Muffin*
Dinner	Asian Fish Fillets* Cooked asparagus 1 cooked beet, sliced and chilled	Falafel* ¼ cup (60 mL) low-fat yogurt or soy yogurt Fast and Easy Greek Salad* Cooked lentils	Easy Black Beans* Personal Garden Herb Salad* Steamed cauliflower or braised Brussels sprouts
Nutrient Boosts	Sprinkle 1 tbsp (15 mL) raw walnuts on beet and drizzle with flaxseed oil Sprinkle ½ tsp (2 mL) nutritional yeast on asparagus	Sprinkle 1 tbsp (15 mL) raw nuts and 2 tsp (10 mL) flaxseed oil on lunch salad	Drizzle 1 tsp (5 mL) flaxseed oil on cauliflower and sprinkle with smoked paprika and ½ tsp (2 mL) nutritional yeast

* The recipe is in the book; unless otherwise indicated, the amount is one serving.

Thursday	Friday	Saturday	Sunday
Hard-cooked egg Legume Guacamole* Carrot, bell pepper and broccoli pieces Cinnamon Tea*	Hard-cooked egg Sardine and Pesto Spread* 2 high-fiber whole-grain crackers Watermelon slice Elderberry Tea*	Raspberry Yogurt Smoothie* 1 apple Flor de Jamaica Tea*	Kitchen Sink Frittata* 1/2 cup (125 mL) sliced strawberries 1/2 cup (125 mL) sliced banana Summer Tea*
1 plum or apple Prickly Pear Power Punch*	1 cooked beet, sliced, chilled and drizzled with 1 tsp (5 mL) lemon juice Prickly Pear Power Punch*	5 canned smoked mussels 2 high-fiber whole-grain crackers Prickly Pear Power Punch*	1/2 cup (125 mL) soy nuts 1/4 cup (60 mL) dried cherries Prickly Pear Power Punch*
Chicken and Bean Salad* Watermelon slice	Kitchen Sink Frittata* 1 cup (250 mL) grapes	Bulgur and Vegetable Lettuce Wraps* 1/2 apple 1 oz (30 g) sharp (old) Cheddar cheese slices	Quick Roasted Red Pepper Dip* Mushrooms, red bell pepper and cherry tomatoes
Sparkling Aloe Hibiscus Spritzer* 1/2 cup (125 mL) raw almonds	Fruit Vinegar Spritzer*	5 figs 1/4 cup (60 mL) raw walnuts Prickly Pear Power Punch*	Spicy Tomato Juice* Baby carrots
Stir-Fried Tofu with Vegetables* Bitter Greens with Paprika* 1 cup (250 mL) cooked brown rice or quinoa	Thai Turkey Stir-Fry* Fried Chinese Mushrooms* Cooked Brussels sprouts, broccoli or asparagus spears	Pan-Seared Mahi Mahi with Papaya Mint Relish* Steamed greens (collards, mustard, kale, Swiss chard) Golden Mushroom Sauté*	Salmon Medallions with Two Purées* Roasted carrots or cauliflower Red Leaf Salad with Mango Chutney Dressing*
Sprinkle 1/4 tsp (1 mL) brewer's yeast and 1 tbsp (15 mL) raw nuts on stir-fry Stir 1 tsp (5 mL) each nutritional yeast and flaxseed oil into quinoa	Sprinkle 1 tsp (5 mL) each raw nuts and ground flax seeds on beet.	Sprinkle 1/2 tsp (2 mL) each nutritional yeast and sesame seeds and 1 tsp (5 mL) flaxseed oil on greens	Sprinkle 1/2 tsp (2 mL) ground flax seeds on carrots Sprinkle 1 tsp (5 mL) flaxseed oil on salad

❧ *Week 4*

	Monday	Tuesday	Wednesday
Breakfast	Raspberry Hibiscus Smoothie* Hard-cooked egg Hibiscus Herb Tea*	Piquant White Bean and Parsley Dip* Sliced bell pepper, zucchini, carrots, and/or cucumber Medicinal Mint Tea*	Carrot Cranberry Muffin* ½ cup (125 mL) low-fat cottage cheese Carrot sticks and bell pepper slices Astragalus Tea*
Snack	Baby carrots ¼ cup (60 mL) raw almonds Prickly Pear Power Punch*	Pineapple Coconut Maca Flax Smoothie*	½ cup (125 mL) blueberries Prickly Pear Power Punch*
Lunch	Cilantro Bean Soup* ½ tart apple 1 oz (30 g) sharp (old) Cheddar cheese slices	Bulgur and Vegetable Lettuce Wraps* Hard-cooked egg ½ oz (15 g) cheese slices or ½ cup (125 mL) low-fat cottage cheese	Country Lentil Soup* 1 oz (30 g) cheese slices
Snack	Red bell pepper slices ¼ cup (60 mL) raw green pumpkin seeds (pepitas) Prickly Pear Power Punch*	¼ cup (60 mL) soy nuts ¼ cup (60 mL) unsweetened dried blueberries Prickly Pear Power Punch*	Minty Lemon Water* 3 to 4 radishes 2 figs
Dinner	Pepper-Crusted Rainbow Trout* Braised Red Cabbage* Spicy Bean Salad*	Mexican Pie* Marinated Vegetable Salad* Grilled zucchini	Grilled Salmon, Mango and Raspberry Spinach Salad* Italian Broiled Tomatoes* Baked winter squash
Nutrient Boosts	Sprinkle 1 tbsp (15 mL) raw nuts on fish and cabbage Drizzle ½ tsp (2 mL) flaxseed oil on bean salad	Stir ¼ tsp (1 mL) brewer's yeast into bean dip Sprinkle 1 tbsp (15 mL) raw nuts and 1 to 2 tsp (5 to 10 mL) flaxseed oil on zucchini	Sprinkle 1 tbsp (15 mL) raw nuts and 1 tsp (5 mL) flaxseed oil on squash

* The recipe is in the book; unless otherwise indicated, the amount is one serving.

Thursday	Friday	Saturday	Sunday
Icy Banana Cashew Smoothie* Cinnamon Tea*	Banana Mango Hibiscus Smoothie* Elderberry Tea*	Country Lentil Soup* ½ apple 1 oz (30 g) sharp (old) Cheddar cheese slices 2 high-fiber whole-grain crackers Flor de Jamaica Tea*	Crustless Zucchini Quiche* Summer Tea*
½ cup (125 mL) black cherries Prickly Pear Power Punch*	Carrot sticks 5 raw Brazil nuts Prickly Pear Power Punch*	4 figs ¼ cup (60 mL) Spanish peanuts Prickly Pear Power Punch*	½ cup (125 mL) blueberries, raspberries or cherries Prickly Pear Power Punch*
Vegetable Quinoa Salad* Roasted Red Pepper and Feta Hummus* Carrot, cucumber and/ or jicama sticks	Cilantro Bean Soup* ½ pear with 1 tsp (5 mL) each crumbled blue cheese and walnuts, and a drizzle of vinaigrette	Mediterranean Lentil and Rice Salad* ½ cup (125 mL) fresh berries Carrot sticks	Curried Butternut Squash and Bean Soup* Red Leaf Salad with Mango Chutney Dressing*
½ cup (125 mL) soy nuts Carrot sticks Prickly Pear Power Punch*	¼ cup (60 mL) soy nuts ¼ cup (60 mL) raisins Prickly Pear Power Punch*	Orange Water* Hard-cooked egg	Red Grape Slushie* Celery sticks spread with hummus
Chickpea Hot Pot* Bulgur Salad with Broccoli, Radishes and Celery*	Turkey Apple Meatloaf* Roasted Vegetables* Sautéed kale, collard greens or bok choy	Chickpea Curry* Sautéed Spinach with Pine Nuts* 1 cup (250 mL) shredded carrots and beets dressed with flax seed oil and herbal vinegar	Poached Fish Jardinière* Orange Broccoli* Mediterranean Lentil and Rice Salad*
Sprinkle 1 tbsp (15 mL) raw nuts on salad, and dress with flaxseed oil	Sprinkle 1 tbsp (15 mL) raw nuts on roasted vegetables Sprinkle 1 tsp (5 mL) each minced garlic, nutritional yeast and flaxseed oil on kale	Sprinkle ½ to 1 tsp (2 to 5 mL) each ground flax seeds and nutritional yeast on salad, and drizzle with 1 tsp (5 mL) flaxseed oil	Drizzle 1 tsp (5 mL) flaxseed oil over fish and broccoli Stir ¼ tsp (1 mL) brewer's yeast into lentil salad

PCOS Boosts

The recipes in this section provide adequate nutrients to maintain general good health according to standard food guides and nutrition analyses. To these recipes, I have added foods and nutrients that are especially valuable in managing PCOS. These PCOS nutritional boosts include the following food groups, food items and food supplements:

Food Groups

- Foods high in quality protein
- Carbohydrate foods that are low on the glycemic index
- Foods high in fiber
- Foods high in essential fatty acids

Food Items

- Legumes
- Lecithin
- Brewer's yeast
- Maca powder
- Ground flax seeds (flaxseed meal)
- Nut flour
- Stevia (*Stevia rebaudiana*) powder and leaf
- Hibiscus (*Hibiscus sabdariffa*) tea
- Prickly pear cactus (*Opuntia ficus-indica*) juice

Food Supplements

- *D-chiro-inositol*
- Chromium
- Magnesium
- Antioxidants (vitamin C, vitamin E and selenium)
- Vitamin D

For more information on the role of these foods and nutrients in managing PCOS, see Parts 1, 2 and 3.

Healthy Starts, Dips and Spreads

Kitchen Sink Frittata

Makes 6 servings

Here's a breakfast recipe that uses leftover cooked vegetables to give you a nutritious start to your day. The golden color of this baked dish is enticing.

Tips

Try using any one or a combination of: mushrooms, broccoli, rapini, fennel, spinach, green peas, green onions, red, green or yellow bell pepper, bok choy, kale, corn, asparagus or green beans. These vegetables are relatively low on the glycemic index.

Choose a full-flavored cheese such as old Cheddar, Gruyère, feta or pepper Jack. The stronger the flavor of the cheese, the less you need to use to get great taste.

All green veggies are naturally high in magnesium, a great nutrient for managing PCOS by improving blood pressure and blood sugar regulation.

Variation

Omit the cheese for a lower-fat dish.

- Preheat oven to 350°F (180°C)
- 8-cup (2 L) baking dish, greased

6	eggs	6
1/2 cup	milk	125 mL
1/4 tsp	salt	1 mL
1/4 tsp	freshly ground black pepper	1 mL
1 tbsp	vegetable oil	15 mL
1/2 cup	diced onion	125 mL
1	sweet potato, peeled and shredded	1
1	tomato, diced	1
2 cups	cooked chopped vegetables (see tip, at left)	500 mL
1 cup	shredded reduced-fat cheese (see tip, at left)	250 mL

1. In a small bowl, whisk eggs and milk. Add salt and pepper. Set aside.

2. In a large skillet, heat oil over medium heat. Sauté onion until softened, about 5 minutes. Stir in sweet potato, tomato and cooked vegetables.

3. Transfer vegetable mixture to prepared baking dish. Pour in egg mixture and top with cheese.

4. Bake in preheated oven for 20 to 30 minutes or until topping is golden and puffed and a knife inserted in the center comes out clean.

PCOS Boost

Boost the chromium and *D-chiro-inositol* content of this recipe by adding 1 tbsp (15 mL) nutritional yeast, 1 tsp (5 mL) brewer's yeast and 1 tsp (5 mL) lecithin to the eggs when whisking them.

Crustless Zucchini Quiche

It's time to make a change. Try starting your day by replacing toast, coffee and dairy products with a baked vegetable quiche and something new to drink: nut milk. Nut milk and nut flour are especially valuable superfoods for managing PCOS symptoms.

Tip

This makes a perfect brunch dish accompanied by a green salad.

Variation

Replace the bread crumbs with a finely ground nut flour, such as almond meal, which is lower than most breads on the glycemic index.

- 9-inch (23 cm) deep-dish pie plate, greased
- Vegetable cooking spray

1 cup	chopped onion	250 mL
5	eggs	5
1½ cups	skim milk	375 mL
2½ cups	grated zucchini, drained	625 mL
2 cups	chopped red bell peppers	500 mL
3 tbsp	all-purpose flour	45 mL
2 tsp	baking powder	10 mL
1 tsp	salt	5 mL
½ tsp	freshly ground black pepper	2 mL
Pinch	cayenne pepper	Pinch
2 cups	shredded light Cheddar cheese	500 mL
¼ cup	dry bread crumbs	60 mL

1. Heat a small frying over medium-high heat. Spray with vegetable cooking spray. Sauté onion until just softened, about 5 minutes.

2. In a large bowl, beat eggs and milk. Stir in onion, zucchini and red peppers.

3. In a small bowl, combine flour, baking powder, salt, black pepper and cayenne. Stir in cheese until thoroughly coated. Add to egg mixture along with bread crumbs. Pour mixture into prepared pie plate and smooth top.

4. Bake in preheated oven for 40 to 50 minutes or until top is lightly browned and puffed and a knife inserted in the center comes out clean.

PCOS Boost

Boost the nutrition of this recipe by adding 1 tbsp (15 mL) lecithin, 1 tbsp (15 mL) nutritional yeast and 1 tsp (5 mL) brewer's yeast, dulse flakes or kelp powder to the eggs when whisking them.

Banana Breakfast Loaf

Makes 14 slices

Here is a popular quick bread recipe, with a twist. Take care to eat just 1 small piece with a high-protein food, such as hard-cooked eggs, leftover fish or a bean soup.

Tips

After you make this loaf, let it cool, wrap it and let it stand overnight to allow the flavors to develop. If you keep the loaf longer than 2 days, store it in the refrigerator.

Do not overmix the batter in step 2. It should be rough or lumpy and stiff.

You will find unsweetened coconut in health food stores and some grocery stores. It is high in saturated fat, so is best used in small quantities.

Be sure to use a high-quality vegetable oil, such as olive or walnut oil.

Variation

Increase the fiber content by adding $\frac{1}{4}$ cup (60 mL) nut flour to the flour mixture or by folding in $\frac{1}{4}$ cup (60 mL) grated carrots or chopped fruit at the end of step 2.

- Preheat oven to 350°F (180°C)
- 8- by 4-inch (20 by 10 cm) metal loaf pan, lightly greased

1½ cups	whole wheat flour	375 mL
½ cup	unsweetened shredded coconut	125 mL
2 tsp	baking powder	10 mL
½ tsp	baking soda	2 mL
½ tsp	salt	2 mL
1 cup	mashed ripe bananas	250 mL
3 tbsp	vegetable oil	45 mL
2 tbsp	liquid honey	30 mL

1. In a large bowl, combine flour, coconut, baking powder, baking soda and salt.

2. In a small bowl, combine banana, oil and honey until well blended. Stir into flour mixture quickly but gently until just blended.

3. Spread batter evenly in prepared loaf pan. Bake in preheated oven for 45 to 50 minutes or until a tester inserted in the center comes out clean. Let cool in pan on a wire rack for 10 minutes, then transfer to the rack to cool completely. Wrap in waxed paper and let stand overnight before slicing.

PCOS Boost

Boost the nutrition of this recipe by replacing $\frac{1}{2}$ cup (125 mL) of the flour with an equal amount of chickpea flour, and adding 1 tbsp (15 mL) lecithin and 1 tsp (5 mL) brewer's yeast to the flour mixture.

Pumpkin Millet Muffins

Makes 12 muffins		

Pumpkins are high in beta carotene and yield delicious, moist muffins. Be sure to use a quality, heat-stable vegetable oil, such as olive or walnut oil. Eat only ½ to 1 of these gluten-free muffins a day, combined with plenty of fresh vegetables and a high-quality protein, such as eggs, beans, or fish.

Tips

If you substitute pumpkin pie spice for the cinnamon, cloves and nutmeg, watch for hidden gluten.

Purchase unroasted, unsalted pumpkin seeds.

Freeze the muffins and thaw just a couple at a time, taking care to eat only 1 or 2 per week.

Variations

Substitute plain yogurt for the sour cream.

For a lower-fat, lactose-free option, replace the milk with nut milk or soy milk, and replace the sour cream with soy yogurt.

- **12-cup muffin tin, lightly greased**

¾ cup	sorghum flour	175 mL
¾ cup	whole bean flour	175 mL
¼ cup	tapioca starch	60 mL
1½ tsp	xanthan gum	7 mL
2 tsp	GF baking powder	10 mL
1 tsp	baking soda	5 mL
½ tsp	salt	2 mL
½ tsp	ground cinnamon	2 mL
¼ tsp	ground cloves	1 mL
¼ tsp	ground nutmeg	1 mL
½ cup	millet seeds	125 mL
¾ cup	green pumpkin seeds, toasted	175 mL
2	eggs	2
1 cup	pumpkin purée (not pie filling)	250 mL
½ cup	milk	125 mL
½ cup	GF sour cream	125 mL
⅓ cup	liquid honey	75 mL
¼ cup	vegetable oil	60 mL

1. In a large bowl or plastic bag, combine sorghum flour, whole bean flour, tapioca starch, xanthan gum, baking powder, baking soda, salt, cinnamon, cloves, nutmeg, millet seeds and pumpkin seeds. Mix well and set aside.

2. In a separate bowl, using an electric mixer, beat eggs, pumpkin purée, milk, sour cream, honey and oil until combined. Add dry ingredients and mix until just combined.

3. Spoon batter evenly into prepared muffin cups. Let stand for 30 minutes. Meanwhile, preheat oven to 350°F (180°C).

4. Bake for 18 to 20 minutes or until firm to the touch. Remove from pan immediately and let cool completely on a rack.

Carrot Cranberry Muffins

Makes 12 muffins

This gluten-free recipe can help satisfy a craving for bread and sweets, but take care to eat only ½ to 1 muffin at any one time, and only in combination with plenty of protein and fresh vegetables. The tart cranberries and orange zest make these muffins taste delightfully fresh, just right to start the day.

Tips

Dried cranberries are often soaked in sugar — not ideal for your dietary goals. Shop for unsweetened dried cranberries or substitute fresh cranberries.

Shred the carrots just before using; exposure to air causes them to darken.

Freeze the muffins and thaw just a couple at a time, taking care to eat only 1 or 2 per week.

Variations

Add ½ cup (125 mL) raisins or chopped walnuts with the cranberries.

Substitute quinoa flour for the teff flour.

- 12-cup muffin tin, lightly greased

1⅓ cups	sorghum flour	325 mL
¼ cup	teff flour	60 mL
¼ cup	tapioca starch	60 mL
1½ tsp	xanthan gum	7 mL
1 tbsp	GF baking powder	15 mL
½ tsp	baking soda	2 mL
½ tsp	salt	2 mL
¾ tsp	ground allspice	3 mL
1 cup	dried cranberries	250 mL
2	eggs	2
1½ cups	shredded carrots	375 mL
2 tbsp	grated orange zest	30 mL
¾ cup	freshly squeezed orange juice	175 mL
⅓ cup	liquid honey	75 mL
¼ cup	vegetable oil	60 mL

1. In a large bowl or plastic bag, combine sorghum flour, teff flour, tapioca starch, xanthan gum, baking powder, baking soda, salt, allspice and cranberries. Mix well and set aside.

2. In a separate bowl, using an electric mixer, beat eggs, carrots, orange zest, orange juice, honey and oil until combined. Add dry ingredients and mix until just combined.

3. Spoon batter evenly into prepared muffin cups. Let stand for 30 minutes. Meanwhile, preheat oven to 350°F (180°C).

4. Bake for 18 to 20 minutes or until firm to the touch. Remove from pan immediately and let cool completely on a rack.

PCOS Boost

Boost the chromium and *D-chiro-inositol* content of this recipe by adding 1 tsp (5 mL) each lecithin and brewer's yeast to the flour mixture.

Spinach Feta Muffins

Makes 12 muffins

These savory gluten-free muffins will awaken your taste buds. They make a great breakfast combined with fish or hard-cooked eggs.

Variation

Use fresh spinach rather than frozen and substitute dulse powder for the salt.

- **12-cup muffin tin, lightly greased**

1	package (10 oz/300 g) frozen spinach	1
1¼ cups	sorghum flour	300 mL
½ cup	quinoa flour	125 mL
⅓ cup	tapioca starch	75 mL
2 tbsp	packed brown sugar	30 mL
1½ tsp	xanthan gum	7 mL
1 tbsp	GF baking powder	15 mL
¼ tsp	salt	1 mL
2 tsp	dried oregano	10 mL
2	eggs	2
1 cup	water	250 mL
3 tbsp	vegetable oil	45 mL
1 tsp	cider vinegar	5 mL
1 cup	snipped dry-packed sun-dried tomatoes	250 mL
½ cup	cubed feta cheese	125 mL

1. In a microwave-safe bowl, defrost spinach on High for 1 minute. Break apart and defrost on High for 1 to 2 minutes or until thawed. Drain and squeeze out excess moisture. Coarsely chop and set aside.

2. In a large bowl or plastic bag, combine sorghum flour, quinoa flour, tapioca starch, brown sugar, xanthan gum, baking powder, salt and oregano. Mix well and set aside.

3. In a separate bowl, using an electric mixer, beat eggs, water, oil, vinegar and spinach until combined. Add dry ingredients and mix until just combined. Stir in sun-dried tomatoes and feta.

4. Spoon batter evenly into prepared muffin cups. Let stand for 30 minutes. Meanwhile, preheat oven to 350°F (180°C).

5. Bake for 22 to 25 minutes or until firm to the touch. Remove from pan immediately and serve warm.

Piquant Marinated Vegetables

Low glycemic load vegetables make a great snack or side dish. All vegetables are good sources of fiber, which helps lower cholesterol and blunts the rise in blood sugar after meals.

Tips

This can be served as a first course salad on leaf lettuce or as a side salad to a meat entrée as well as an appetizer. Make the entire recipe. It improves with time and keeps very well.

When purchasing cauliflower or broccoli, take note of the smell. If these vegetables have passed their peak, they will have a strong, unpleasant odor.

The sugar in the marinade is not essential and may be omitted or replaced with stevia powder.

2 cups	cauliflower florets	500 mL
2 cups	broccoli florets	500 mL
1 cup	mushrooms	250 mL
½	red bell pepper, cut into strips	½
1 cup	cut-up green beans	250 mL
8	small white pickling onions	8
1	carrot, cut into rounds	1
	Lettuce leaves	
	Cherry tomatoes and chopped fresh parsley	

Marinade

1 cup	red wine vinegar	250 mL
1 tsp	dried oregano	5 mL
1 tsp	dried tarragon	5 mL
½ tsp	granulated sugar	2 mL
½ tsp	salt	2 mL
¼ tsp	freshly ground black pepper	1 mL
¼ cup	olive oil	60 mL

1. In a bowl, combine cauliflower, broccoli, mushrooms, red pepper, green beans, onions and carrot.

2. *Marinade:* In a saucepan, heat vinegar and seasonings; add oil and pour over vegetables. Cool slightly and transfer mixture to a large plastic bag. Refrigerate for 24 hours before serving.

3. Serve in bowl lined with lettuce; garnish with cherry tomatoes and parsley. Provide toothpicks for spearing vegetables.

PCOS Boost

Boost the nutrition of this recipe by sprinkling the vegetables with dulse flakes and nutritional yeast before serving.

Grilled Stuffed Jalapeño Peppers

Makes 4 servings	

These peppers are hot, hot, hot, but delicious when combined with hummus and grilled. Beans, such as the chickpeas in hummus, help balance blood sugar and cholesterol, and their inositol improves insulin reception in cells. Hot peppers improve circulation and may improve cholesterol levels.

Tip

Wear disposable gloves when working with jalapeños so the hot oils do not touch your skin.

Variation

In place of the hummus, stuff peppers with a mixture of ¼ cup (60 mL) light cream cheese, 2 tsp (10 mL) finely minced shallots, 2 tsp (10 mL) freshly squeezed lime juice, 1 tsp (5 mL) finely minced garlic and ¼ tsp (1 mL) freshly ground black pepper.

- Preheat barbecue grill to medium

4	jalapeño peppers, halved lengthwise and seeded	4
¼ cup	chile pepper–flavored hummus or other hummus	60 mL

1. Fill each jalapeño half with $1\frac{1}{2}$ tsp (7 mL) hummus. Place on preheated barbecue, filling side up, and grill for 4 to 5 minutes or until grill marks form on underside of pepper.

PCOS Boost

Boost the chromium and *D-chiro-inositol* content of this recipe by stirring 1 tsp (5 mL) each brewer's yeast, nutritional yeast and lecithin into the hummus before filling the peppers. To increase the protein and healthy fats, sprinkle the grilled peppers with crushed almonds or cashews before serving.

Lentil-Stuffed Tomatoes

Lentils are PCOS superfoods, and when stuffed in tomatoes and baked, they are also super-delicious. Consider making legumes your number one source of protein.

Tips

Prepare these tomatoes to serve as a side dish with oven-cooked meals. They can be stuffed up to 4 hours in advance, refrigerated, then heated (allow a longer heating time in this case).

The amount of salt in canned legumes varies from brand to brand, so be sure to check the sodium value in the Nutrition Facts table. Draining and rinsing the beans before use removes about 50% of the sodium.

- **Preheat oven to 400°F (200°C)**
- **6- or 12-cup muffin pan**

4	firm tomatoes	4
¼ cup	finely chopped celery	60 mL
1 tbsp	finely chopped onion	15 mL
1 tbsp	finely chopped green bell pepper	15 mL
½ tsp	curry powder	2 mL
1 cup	rinsed drained canned brown lentils	250 mL
1 tbsp	freshly grated Parmesan cheese	15 mL

1. Core tomatoes and cut a thin slice from the top of each. Scoop pulp and juice into a skillet and mash pulp. Place tomato shells cut side down on a paper towel to drain.

2. Add celery, onion, green pepper and curry powder to tomato pulp and juice. Cook, stirring, over medium heat for about 5 minutes or until vegetables are tender. Add lentils and cook, stirring, until mixture is thickened.

3. Spoon lentil mixture into tomato shells. Sprinkle with Parmesan. Place stuffed tomatoes in 4 muffin cups. Set muffin pan on a baking sheet.

4. Bake in preheated oven for 10 minutes or until heated through.

PCOS Boost

Boost the nutrition of this recipe by adding 1 tsp (5 mL) each brewer's yeast, lecithin and nutritional yeast to the lentil mixture. Sprinkle each stuffed tomato with dulse powder and sesame seeds.

Scalloped Soybeans

Makes 6 servings

A variation on scalloped potatoes, this recipe features soybeans, which, like other legumes, help stabilize blood sugar and cholesterol levels. Enjoy them often!

Variations

Substitute 3 cups (750 mL) rinsed drained canned soybeans for the dried. Skip steps 1 and 2.

To reduce the glycemic load, substitute nut flour and nutritional yeast for the bread crumbs.

- **6-cup (1.5 L) casserole dish**

1 cup	dried soybeans, rinsed	250 mL
1	onion, chopped	1
1 cup	chopped celery	250 mL
½ cup	finely chopped red or green bell pepper	125 mL
½ tsp	salt	2 mL
½ cup	no-salt-added tomato sauce	125 mL
¼ cup	boiling water	60 mL
¼ cup	fresh bread crumbs	60 mL
2 tsp	olive oil	10 mL

1. Place soybeans in a large bowl and add enough cold water to cover by at least 3 inches (7.5 cm). Cover and let stand at room temperature for at least 12 hours or for up to 24 hours.

2. Drain soybeans and rinse well; drain. In a saucepan, combine soybeans and 3 cups (750 mL) fresh water. Bring to a boil over high heat and boil for 10 minutes. Reduce heat to low, cover and simmer for 1½ to 2 hours or until soybeans are softened. Drain.

3. Meanwhile, preheat oven to 350°F (180°C).

4. Pour soybeans into casserole dish. Stir in onion, celery, red pepper, salt, tomato sauce and boiling water.

5. In a bowl, combine bread crumbs and oil. Sprinkle over soybean mixture.

6. Bake in preheated oven for 1½ to 2 hours or until soybeans are tender.

PCOS Boost

Boost the chromium and *D-chiro-inositol* content of this recipe by stirring 1 tsp (5 mL) each lecithin and brewer's yeast into the soybean mixture.

Lemon Pesto Sauce

Makes about ⅓ cup (75 mL)		

This zesty homemade pesto makes a great substitute for store-bought dips and spreads. Spread it on fish or use it as a dip with raw vegetable slices.

Tip

When fresh basil is not available, replace with 1 cup (250 mL) fresh parsley leaves and 2 tbsp (30 mL) dried basil.

- **Food processor or blender**

1 cup	packed fresh basil leaves (see tip, at left)	250 mL
1	clove garlic	1
1 tbsp	olive oil	15 mL
1 tbsp	almonds or pine nuts	15 mL
4 tsp	freshly squeezed lemon juice	20 mL
1 tsp	grated lemon zest	5 mL

1. In food processor, combine basil, garlic, oil, almonds, lemon juice and zest. Blend until coarsely chopped. Chill or freeze, as desired.

PCOS Boost

Boost the nutrition of this recipe by adding 1 tsp (5 mL) each brewer's yeast and lecithin.

Pico de Gallo

Makes 8 servings		

Having flavorful dips and spreads on hand can help you do without high glycemic breads and snack foods. Enjoy this salsa with a variety of raw vegetable slices and bean dips. Besides being delicious, hot herbs and spices, such as garlic and hot peppers, have beneficial effects on blood sugar and cholesterol.

1	clove garlic, finely chopped	1
2 cups	chopped seeded tomatoes	500 mL
1 cup	diced Spanish onion	250 mL
½ cup	minced fresh cilantro	125 mL
1 tbsp	minced seeded jalapeño pepper	15 mL
1 tbsp	freshly squeezed lime juice	15 mL
½ tsp	salt	2 mL

1. In a medium bowl, combine garlic, tomatoes, onion, cilantro, jalapeño, lime juice and salt. Cover and refrigerate for at least 1 hour or overnight to allow flavors to meld.

Black Bean Salsa

Makes 8 servings

Enjoy this salsa on top of refried beans or a cooked whole grain, such as quinoa, or serve as a dip with raw vegetable slices. Vegetables are rich sources of antioxidant nutrients and magnesium, needed to balance the hormones involved in PCOS.

Tip

If your family does not like heat, cut back on the amount of jalapeño or omit it.

3	tomatoes, diced	3
1	small red onion, finely chopped	1
1	jalapeño pepper, ribs and seeds removed, finely chopped	1
1	can (19 oz/540 mL) black beans, drained and rinsed (about 2 cups/500 mL)	1
½ cup	chopped fresh cilantro	125 mL
1 tbsp	olive oil	15 mL
½ tsp	salt	2 mL
	Juice of 2 limes	

1. In a large bowl, combine tomatoes, red onion, jalapeño, beans, cilantro, olive oil, salt and lime juice. Cover and refrigerate for at least 2 hours or overnight to allow flavors to meld.

PCOS Boost

Boost the chromium content of this recipe by substituting dulse flakes for the salt and adding ½ tsp (2 mL) brewer's yeast.

Legume Guacamole

<table>
<tr><td colspan="2">Makes about
1½ cups (375 mL)</td></tr>
</table>

Avocados offer "good" fats and are high in vitamin E. All of the spices in this recipe help lower cholesterol and support the cardiovascular system. The salt may be replaced with dulse powder.

Tips

Vary the heat and flavor intensity by adjusting the amounts of lime juice, jalapeño and hot pepper sauce.

Use this as a spread on grilled vegetable sandwiches.

If you dislike cilantro, use chopped fresh parsley instead.

Variation

To reduce the fat content of this recipe, omit the mayonnaise or substitute nonfat plain yogurt.

• **Food processor or blender**

1 cup	frozen baby peas	250 mL
1	ripe avocado	1
3	cloves garlic, minced	3
1	jalapeño pepper, seeded and coarsely chopped	1
¼ cup	coarsely chopped fresh cilantro	60 mL
2 tbsp	chopped red onion	30 mL
3 tbsp	freshly squeezed lime or lemon juice	45 mL
2 tbsp	light mayonnaise	30 mL
1 tsp	ground cumin	5 mL
½ tsp	chili powder	2 mL
½ tsp	freshly ground white pepper	2 mL
¼ tsp	salt	1 mL
1 cup	coarsely chopped plum (Roma) tomatoes	250 mL
½ to 1 tsp	hot pepper sauce (optional)	2 to 5 mL

1. In a small saucepan, bring ¼ cup (60 mL) water to a boil over high heat. Add peas and return to a boil. Reduce heat to low, cover and simmer for 4 minutes. Remove from heat and let cool.

2. Peel avocado and scoop flesh into food processor. Add cooled peas (along with any remaining liquid from the pan), garlic, jalapeño, cilantro, red onion, lime juice, mayonnaise, cumin, chili powder, pepper and salt; pulse until chopped. Purée for about 1 minute or until mostly smooth with some small bits remaining.

3. Transfer to a bowl and gently stir in tomatoes. Season to taste with hot pepper sauce (if using).

PCOS Boost

Boost the nutrition of this recipe by adding 2 tsp (10 mL) lecithin and 1 tsp (5 mL) brewer's yeast before puréeing.

Yogurt Dill Dip with Belgian Endive

	Makes about 2 cups (500 mL)	

Did you know that you can make a low-fat cheese from yogurt? For a salty, flavorful version, add dulse flakes when draining the yogurt.

Tips

For the best texture, when choosing yogurt for this recipe, read the label carefully and make sure it doesn't contain any gelatin or starch.

You can let the yogurt drain for up to 1 day. The longer it drains, the thicker it will become.

This dip would make a delicious topping for grilled chicken.

- Colander or strainer
- Cheesecloth

3 cups	low-fat plain yogurt (see tip, at left)	750 mL
1	clove garlic, finely minced	1
2 tbsp	chopped fresh dill	30 mL
¼ tsp	salt	1 mL
¼ tsp	freshly ground white pepper	1 mL
1 tsp	extra virgin olive oil or canola oil	5 mL
	Grated zest and juice of 1 lemon	
2	heads Belgian endive, leaves separated	2

1. Line colander with a double layer of cheesecloth and set over a large bowl. Place yogurt in colander, cover and refrigerate. Let drain for 3 to 5 hours or until yogurt is thickened and resembles soft cream cheese. Discard liquid in bowl.

2. Place yogurt cheese in a medium bowl. Stir in garlic, dill, salt, pepper, oil, lemon zest and lemon juice. Serve with endive leaves for dipping.

PCOS Boost

Boost the nutrition of this recipe by sprinkling the endive leaves with nutritional yeast and freshly ground nut flour. Add 1 tsp (5 mL) lecithin and ½ tsp (2 mL) brewer's yeast to the yogurt mixture.

Quick Roasted Red Pepper Dip

Makes 6 servings		

Every home chef needs a recipe for a basic red pepper dip, and this one is especially rich in flavor and nutrients.

Tips

Serve this delicious dip with raw vegetables, whole wheat pita triangles or whole wheat crackers.

Roasted red peppers are flavorful and offer key nutrients. No wonder they often appear as an ingredient in recipes. You can roast them yourself and freeze them for later use or purchase them already prepared in a jar.

Variations

If you like garlic, increase the garlic to 2 or 3 cloves.

To increase the healthy fat content in this recipe, stir in $1/4$ cup (60 mL) crushed raw nuts before chilling.

- **Food processor or blender**

3	roasted red bell peppers	3
$3/4$ cup	feta cheese, drained and crumbled (about 6 oz/175 g)	175 mL
$1/2$ tsp	minced garlic	2 mL
$1/4$ tsp	hot pepper flakes	1 mL

1. In food processor, purée peppers, feta cheese, garlic and hot pepper flakes. Chill before serving.

PCOS Boost

Boost the nutrition of this recipe by adding 1 tsp (5 mL) lecithin and $1/2$ tsp (2 mL) brewer's yeast.

Roasted Red Pepper and Feta Hummus

<table>
<tr><td colspan="3">• Food processor or blender</td></tr>
</table>

Makes about 2 cups (500 mL)

If you love hummus, try this old standard with a healthy twist. The chickpeas and spices help balance blood sugar levels. Enjoy this with raw veggies that are low on the glycemic index.

2	roasted red bell peppers	2
2	cloves garlic, minced	2
1	can (19 oz/540 mL) chickpeas, drained and rinsed (about 2 cups/500 mL)	1
1/2 cup	crumbled feta cheese	125 mL
2 tbsp	chopped fresh parsley	30 mL
2 tbsp	tahini	30 mL
2 tbsp	freshly squeezed lemon juice	30 mL
1 tbsp	canola oil	15 mL
1/4 tsp	cayenne pepper	1 mL
1/2	lemon	1/2

1. In food processor, combine roasted peppers, garlic, chickpeas, feta, parsley, tahini, 2 tbsp (30 mL) lemon juice, 2 tbsp (30 mL) water, oil and cayenne; process until smooth.

2. Transfer to a bowl, cover and refrigerate for at least 1 hour, until chilled, or for up to 1 day. Squeeze fresh lemon juice over dip before serving.

Tips

Tahini is a paste or butter made from crushed sesame seeds. It has a distinctive nutty taste and coarse texture. It is frequently used in Middle Eastern cooking.

Try using an immersion blender to process the ingredients.

Serve with an assortment of fresh vegetables.

Variation

Substitute unsweetened natural peanut butter for the tahini, provided no one at the table has a nut allergy.

PCOS Boost

Boost the chromium and *D-chiro-inositol* content of this recipe by adding 1 tsp (5 mL) lecithin and 1/2 tsp (2 mL) brewer's yeast.

Spicy Hummus

Here's a sharper-tasting hummus. Beans offer a good deal of protein and can be enjoyed not only for starters and snacks, but also for breakfast. Serve with raw veggie slices for dipping or make a vegetable "sandwich" using tomato and cucumber rounds instead of bread.

Tips

If the hummus is too thick for your taste, blend in a little water.

Hummus will keep for up to 1 week in the refrigerator.

Serve hummus in a hollowed-out red pepper for a nice presentation when entertaining.

- **Blender or food processor**

1	can (19 oz/540 mL) chickpeas, drained and rinsed (about 2 cups/500 mL)	1
2	cloves garlic	2
1/4 tsp	ground cumin	1 mL
1/4 tsp	ground coriander	1 mL
1/4 tsp	hot pepper sauce	1 mL
1 tbsp	freshly squeezed lemon juice	15 mL

1. In blender or food processor, on medium speed, blend chickpeas, garlic, cumin, coriander and hot pepper sauce for 30 seconds or until finely chopped. Add lemon juice and blend until smooth.

PCOS Boost

Boost the chromium and *D-chiro-inositol* content of this recipe by adding 1 tsp (5 mL) lecithin and 1/2 tsp (2 mL) brewer's yeast.

Piquant White Bean and Parsley Dip

<table>
<tr><td colspan="3">Makes about 1½ cups (375 mL)</td></tr>
</table>

Here's another delicious way to get your daily legumes. Spread this piquant dip on roasted eggplant, zucchini, onions and peppers. Try it for breakfast.

Tip

It's best to start by adding just 1 pepper to the dip, then you can add more to taste.

Variation

For Asian flair, add a few drops of sesame oil and garnish this dip with sesame seeds.

- **Food processor or blender**

2	green onions, coarsely chopped	2
2	cloves garlic, minced	2
1 to 2	jalapeño peppers, seeded and coarsely chopped	1 to 2
1	can (19 oz/540 mL) white kidney beans, drained and rinsed (about 2 cups/500 mL)	1
½ cup	loosely packed chopped fresh parsley	125 mL
¼ cup	freshly squeezed lemon juice	60 mL
1 tbsp	canola oil	15 mL
1 tsp	ground cumin	5 mL

1. In food processor, combine green onions, garlic, jalapeños to taste, beans, parsley, lemon juice, oil and cumin; process until smooth.

2. Transfer to a bowl, cover and refrigerate for at least 1 hour, until chilled, or for up to 1 day.

PCOS Boost

Boost the essential fatty acid content of this recipe by adding ¼ cup (60 mL) raw nuts. For a salty version high in chromium, add 1 tsp (5 mL) dulse flakes.

Sardine and Pesto Spread

This spread is truly original and absolutely delicious. Sardines are rich in essential fatty acids, which help improve cholesterol ratios and support heart health. If serving the spread with crackers or baguette slices, be sure to also load them up with veggies (such as finely grated carrots, minced bell peppers, minced onions and sliced cucumber) to blunt the high glycemic effects of the bread.

Tips

Don't mash the sardines too much, or you'll end up with more of a paste than a spread.

Try Mediterranean-style or lemon-flavored sardines.

Serve with crudités, whole-grain crackers or toasted French baguette slices.

1	can (3½ oz/106 g) sardines, drained	1
2 tbsp	basil pesto	30 mL
1 tbsp	freshly squeezed lime juice	15 mL

1. In a small bowl, mash sardines with a fork. Stir in pesto and lime juice until just blended.

Soups and Sandwiches

Carrot and Ginger Soup

The maple syrup in this recipe makes it a standout, so enjoy it occasionally even though the syrup is high on the glycemic index. Both ginger and garlic have beneficial effects on blood sugar and cholesterol levels. Eat them wherever you can.

Tip

Use the side of a spoon to scrape the skin off gingerroot before chopping or grating. Gingerroot keeps well in the freezer for up to 3 months and can be grated from frozen.

Variations

Substitute almond milk or soy milk for the cow's milk.

Omit the maple syrup or substitute ¼ tsp (1 mL) stevia powder.

- **Blender or food processor**

3 cups	water	750 mL
2	cloves garlic, crushed	2
4 cups	sliced carrots	1 L
½ cup	chopped onion	125 mL
1 tbsp	vegetable bouillon powder	15 mL
2 tsp	pure maple syrup	10 mL
1 tsp	curry powder	5 mL
½ tsp	grated gingerroot	2 mL
1½ cups	milk	375 mL

1. In a large saucepan, bring water to a boil. Add garlic, carrots, onion, bouillon powder, maple syrup, curry powder and ginger; return to a boil. Reduce heat, cover and simmer for 40 to 45 minutes or until carrots are tender. Remove from heat.

2. Working in batches, transfer soup to blender and purée on high speed until smooth.

3. Return soup to saucepan and add milk. Heat over low heat (do not boil or milk will curdle).

PCOS Boost

Boost the nutrition of this recipe by adding 1 tbsp (15 mL) lecithin and 2 tsp (10 mL) each brewer's yeast and nutritional yeast when puréeing the soup.

Roasted Cauliflower and Red Pepper Soup

This delicious soup makes a great alternative breakfast or starter. Cauliflower, like all cruciferous vegetables, is believed to help the body metabolize reproductive hormones — a boon for women with PCOS. The carrots and red peppers make this soup high in antioxidant nutrients.

Tip

Cutting the cauliflower into bite-size florets makes for easy eating.

Variations

Use a combination of cauliflower and broccoli, keeping the total amount at 5 cups (1.25 L).

To make this soup vegan, substitute vegetable broth for the chicken broth.

- Preheat oven to 425°F (220°C)
- Rimmed baking sheet, lined with foil

5 cups	bite-size cauliflower florets	1.25 L
4 tsp	canola oil, divided	20 mL
1 cup	finely chopped onion	250 mL
1 cup	finely chopped carrots	250 mL
2	cloves garlic, minced	2
4 cups	reduced-sodium chicken broth	1 L
2	roasted red bell peppers, finely chopped	2
2	sprigs fresh thyme	2
	Freshly ground black pepper	

1. Place cauliflower on prepared baking sheet and drizzle with 2 tsp (10 mL) of the oil. Roast in preheated oven, turning once, for 20 to 25 minutes or until florets start to caramelize and are lightly browned.

2. Meanwhile, in a large pot, heat the remaining oil over medium heat. Sauté onion and carrots for 3 to 4 minutes or until softened. Add garlic and sauté for 30 seconds. Stir in caramelized cauliflower, broth, roasted peppers and thyme; increase heat to high and bring to a boil. Reduce heat and simmer for 10 minutes to blend the flavors. Discard thyme sprigs. Season to taste with pepper.

PCOS Boost

Boost the nutrition of this recipe by adding 1 tbsp (15 mL) lecithin and 1 tsp (5 mL) brewer's yeast with the broth.

Ginger Soy Mushroom Soup

Mushrooms make great soups and are low on the glycemic index. Serve this Asian-inspired version with a raw salad, for a nutritious meal.

Tips

Be sure to use firm tofu in this soup. Otherwise, it won't retain its shape.

Sesame oil is available in large supermarkets and specialty food shops. All you need is a teaspoon (5 mL) to enhance the flavor of this soup.

5 cups	chicken broth	1.25 L
4 tsp	finely chopped gingerroot	20 mL
8 oz	sliced mushrooms (shiitake, oyster, portobello or a combination), about 2 cups (500 mL)	250 g
2 tbsp	sodium-reduced soy sauce	30 mL
1 tsp	sesame oil	5 mL
8 oz	firm tofu, cut into small cubes	250 g
1	green onion, thinly sliced	1

1. In a saucepan, combine broth, gingerroot and mushrooms; bring to a boil. Reduce heat and simmer, uncovered, for 15 minutes. Stir in soy sauce and sesame oil.

2. Place tofu and green onion in individual soup bowls or tureen. Add soup and serve.

PCOS Boost

Boost the chromium content of this recipe by adding 1 to 2 tsp (5 to 10 mL) each dulse flakes and brewer's yeast.

Caramelized Onion and Roasted Mushroom Soup

Makes 6 servings

This version of mushroom soup features the savory flavors of caramelized onion, rosemary, thyme and Marsala. It's the perfect comfort food on a cold day.

Tips

Marsala is a fortified wine (i.e., it has brandy or another spirit added to it) made from Sicilian grapes.

Be sure to remove the rosemary and thyme sprigs before serving so that there are no hard, woody parts in the soup.

- Preheat oven to 425°F (220°C)
- Rimmed baking sheet

1 lb	mushrooms, quartered	500 g
2 tbsp	canola oil, divided	30 mL
4	sprigs fresh rosemary, divided	4
4	sprigs fresh thyme, divided	4
1 tsp	freshly ground black pepper, divided	5 mL
2 cups	coarsely chopped onions	500 mL
¼ cup	coarsely chopped shallots	60 mL
¼ cup	Marsala wine	60 mL
4 cups	reduced-sodium chicken broth	1 L
1	bay leaf	1

1. Place mushrooms on baking sheet and drizzle with 1 tbsp (15 mL) of the oil. Add 2 sprigs each rosemary and thyme. Sprinkle with ½ tsp (2 mL) pepper. Roast in preheated oven, stirring occasionally, for 20 to 25 minutes or until mushrooms are golden brown. Discard rosemary and thyme sprigs. Set mushrooms aside.

2. Meanwhile, in a large pot, heat the remaining oil over medium heat. Sauté onions and shallots for 2 minutes. Reduce heat to low and cook, stirring frequently, for about 15 minutes or until onions are caramelized (dark golden brown).

3. Add Marsala and deglaze the pot, scraping up any brown bits stuck to the bottom. Add roasted mushrooms, broth, bay leaf and the remaining rosemary, thyme and pepper; increase heat to high and bring to a boil. Reduce heat and simmer for 15 minutes to blend the flavors. Discard rosemary and thyme sprigs and bay leaf.

PCOS Boost

Boost the *D-chiro-inositol* content of this recipe by adding 1 tbsp (15 mL) lecithin and 1 to 2 tsp (5 to 10 mL) brewer's yeast.

Curried Butternut Squash and Bean Soup

This hearty soup has a creamy texture but contains no dairy products, and all the spices help maintain healthy blood fat levels. If you like the flavor of dulse, add 2 tsp (10 mL) when puréeing the soup. If you like garlic, you could use 4 or 5 cloves.

Tips

To make 2 cups (500 mL) mashed cooked butternut squash, use 1 medium squash. Cut it in half lengthwise and scoop out the seeds. Place it cut side down on a lightly greased baking sheet and prick the skin several times with a fork. Bake in a 375°F (190°C) oven for about 30 minutes or until fork-tender. Let cool, then scoop out the flesh and discard the skin. If you have more flesh than you need, reserve the extra for another use.

To reduce the sodium in this soup, look for a reduced-sodium vegetable broth.

- **Food processor, blender or immersion blender**

1 tbsp	canola oil	15 mL
½ cup	coarsely chopped onion	125 mL
½ cup	coarsely chopped carrot	125 mL
½ cup	coarsely chopped celery	125 mL
2	cloves garlic, minced	2
1 tsp	minced gingerroot	5 mL
2 tsp	curry powder	10 mL
1½ tsp	ground cumin	7 mL
1	can (19 oz/540 mL) white kidney beans, drained and rinsed (about 2 cups/500 mL)	1
2 cups	mashed cooked butternut or acorn squash (see tip, at left)	500 mL
2 cups	vegetable broth	500 mL
	Salt and freshly ground black pepper	

1. In a large pot, heat oil over medium high heat. Sauté onion, carrot and celery for 4 to 5 minutes or until softened. Add garlic, ginger, curry powder and cumin; sauté for 30 seconds. Stir in beans, squash, broth and 2 cups (500 mL) water; bring to a boil. Reduce heat and simmer, stirring occasionally, for 30 minutes to blend the flavors.

2. Working in batches, transfer soup to food processor (or use immersion blender in pot) and purée until smooth. Return soup to pot (if necessary) and season to taste with salt and pepper.

PCOS Boost

Boost the nutrition of this recipe by adding 1 tbsp (15 mL) lecithin and 2 tsp (10 mL) each brewer's yeast and nutritional yeast.

Thai-Style Squash Soup

Makes 12 servings

The delicious seasonings make this soup exceptional. It is loaded with garlic, which helps to support healthy blood sugar and cholesterol levels. Squash is high in fiber, rich in anti-inflammatory flavonoids and low on the glycemic index. Eat it more often.

Tips

This recipe is best when squash is in season. You can often find peeled and chopped butternut squash in the produce section of the supermarket. Buy it, as it will save you time and effort: no blisters that way!

For convenience, buy a jar of minced ginger.

If you can't find wild lime leaves locally, substitute grated lime zest (3 leaves = the zest of 1 lime).

If you are lucky enough to have any leftovers, this soup is great as a sauce over grilled fish, chicken or pork.

- Preheat oven to 350°F (180°C)
- Blender or food processor

1	head garlic	1
1 tbsp	olive oil	15 mL
2 tbsp	vegetable oil	30 mL
1	onion, diced	1
2 tbsp	finely minced gingerroot	30 mL
2 tbsp	finely minced lemongrass	30 mL
1	large butternut squash, peeled, seeded and diced	1
3¼ cups	reduced-sodium chicken broth	800 mL
1	can (14 oz/400 mL) light coconut milk	1
	Salt and freshly ground black pepper	
4	wild lime leaves (optional)	4

1. Cut top off head of garlic to expose the cloves. Place on a small piece of foil wrap. Drizzle with olive oil. Cover with foil and bake in preheated oven for 30 minutes or until cloves are soft.

2. Meanwhile, in a large saucepan, heat vegetable oil over medium heat. Sauté onion, ginger and lemongrass until tender, about 5 minutes. Add squash and broth; bring to a boil. Reduce heat, cover and simmer for 30 minutes. Remove from heat. Squeeze roasted garlic into soup, making sure not to get any skin in soup.

3. Working in batches, transfer soup to blender and purée on high speed until smooth.

4. Return soup to saucepan and stir in coconut milk. Season to taste with salt and pepper. Add wild lime leaves, if using. Heat over low heat for 10 minutes or until heated through and lime flavor infuses soup.

PCOS Boost

Boost the nutrition of this recipe by adding 1 tbsp (15 mL) each lecithin and nutritional yeast and 2 tsp (10 mL) brewer's yeast.

Country Lentil Soup

Makes 8 servings

Lentils, like all legumes, are a good source of high-quality protein. They are also a great way to start the day.

Tip

If you prefer, when puréeing soups you can use an immersion blender and blend the soup right in the pot. This will save you some cleanup time, but the result will be less smooth.

Variations

Substitute green lentils, well rinsed and drained, canned chickpeas or white kidney beans for the red lentils. Decrease the simmering time to 15 minutes if using canned legumes.

To make this a heartier soup, add 1 cup (250 mL) diced cooked lean ham after puréeing.

- Blender or food processor

1 tbsp	vegetable oil	15 mL
1 cup	diced onion	250 mL
½ cup	diced carrot	125 mL
½ cup	diced celery	125 mL
4 cups	vegetable or chicken broth	1 L
1 cup	dried red lentils, well rinsed	250 mL
¼ tsp	dried thyme	1 mL
	Salt and freshly ground black pepper	
½ cup	chopped fresh flat-leaf parsley	125 mL

1. In a large saucepan, heat oil over medium heat. Sauté onion, carrot and celery until softened, about 5 minutes. Add broth, lentils and thyme; bring to a boil. Reduce heat, cover and simmer for 20 minutes or until lentils are soft. Remove from heat.

2. Working in batches, transfer soup to blender. Purée on high speed until creamy. Add up to 1 cup (250 mL) water if purée is too thick. Season to taste with salt and pepper. Return to saucepan to reheat, if necessary.

3. Ladle into bowls and garnish with parsley.

PCOS Boost

Boost the chromium and *D-chiro-inositol* content of this recipe by adding 1 tbsp (15 mL) lecithin and 1 tsp (5 mL) each brewer's yeast and nutritional yeast.

Cilantro Bean Soup

Makes 8 servings

The beans and vegetables make this soup a healthy lunch or starter — or even an alternative breakfast. The warm flavors of cilantro and coriander shine through.

Tips

You do not have to blend this soup if you would rather have it chunky.

Vary the beans by substituting black beans, kidney beans or chickpeas.

Variation

For a version that's lower on the glycemic index, substitute sweet potato for the potato.

- **Blender or food processor**

1 tbsp	vegetable oil	15 mL
2	onions, chopped	2
1 cup	diced carrots	250 mL
½ cup	diced celery	125 mL
½ tsp	ground cumin	2 mL
½ tsp	ground coriander	2 mL
1	can (19 oz/540 mL) white beans, drained and rinsed (about 2 cups/500 mL)	1
1	tomato, seeded and chopped	1
3½ cups	reduced-sodium chicken or vegetable broth	875 mL
1 cup	roughly chopped fresh cilantro	250 mL
1 cup	diced peeled potato	250 mL
	Salt and freshly ground black pepper	
	Additional chopped fresh cilantro (optional)	

1. In a large saucepan, heat oil over medium heat. Sauté onions, carrots and celery until softened, about 5 minutes. Stir in cumin and coriander; cook for 1 minute. Add beans, tomato, broth, cilantro, potato, and salt and pepper to taste; bring to a boil. Reduce heat, cover and simmer for 25 minutes or until vegetables are just soft. Remove from heat.

2. Working in batches, transfer soup to blender and purée on high speed until smooth. Return to pot and reheat, if necessary.

3. Ladle into bowls and garnish with cilantro, if desired.

PCOS Boost

Boost the nutrition of this recipe by adding 1 tbsp (15 mL) lecithin and 1 tsp (5 mL) each brewer's and nutritional yeast. Sprinkle with raw sesame seeds, crushed walnuts or other raw nuts at serving time.

Vegetarian Chili

This chili is comfort food at its best. No surprises here — just the flavors you expect from a vegetarian standard.

Tips

If you cannot find Mexican-flavored vegetarian ground round, use regular vegetarian ground round and add 2 tbsp (30 mL) chili powder.

Use a heat-stable oil, such as walnut oil, to sauté the vegetables.

Variations

Use organic, hormone-free ground turkey with several teaspoons of Mexican spice seasoning in place of the vegetarian ground round.

Substitute a 12-oz (341 mL) can of peaches-and-cream corn, drained, for the carrots.

For a lower-fat option, omit the cheese.

1 tbsp	vegetable oil	15 mL
2	cloves garlic, diced	2
1/2 cup	diced red onion	125 mL
1	package (12 oz/340 g) Mexican-flavored vegetarian ground round	1
1 cup	diced green bell pepper	250 mL
2	cans (each 19 oz/540 mL) diced tomatoes (about 4¾ cups/1.175 L)	2
1	can (19 oz/540 mL) red kidney beans, drained and rinsed (about 2 cups/500 mL)	1
1 cup	grated carrots	250 mL
1 tbsp	dried parsley	15 mL
1 tsp	hot pepper sauce	5 mL
	Freshly ground black pepper	
1/2 cup	shredded Cheddar cheese	125 mL

1. In a large skillet, heat oil over medium heat. Sauté garlic and red onion until softened, about 5 minutes. Add ground round, breaking it apart with a wooden spoon to prevent clumps; sauté for 2 to 3 minutes or until evenly heated. Add green pepper and sauté for 2 to 3 minutes. Add tomatoes, beans, carrots, parsley, hot pepper sauce and black pepper to taste; cook, stirring occasionally, for 10 minutes or until beans are heated through.

2. Ladle into serving bowls and sprinkle with cheese.

PCOS Boost

Boost the chromium and *D-chiro-inositol* content of this recipe by adding 1 tbsp (15 mL) lecithin and 2 tsp (10 mL) each brewer's and nutritional yeast.

Veggie Sandwich

Makes 1 serving

This lettuce wrap can be whipped up in a mere minute. Eat several of these instead of bread- or bagel-based sandwiches.

Variation

Substitute low-fat plain yogurt for the cream cheese.

1	piece red leaf lettuce (or lettuce of your choice)	1
1 tsp	cream cheese	5 mL
1	baby carrot, cut into 4 slivers	1

1. Wash lettuce and pat dry. Spread cream cheese on lettuce. Place carrot slivers up the middle of the lettuce on top of the cream cheese. Roll up lettuce.

PCOS Boost

Boost the nutrition of this recipe by adding minced garlic, onion or other raw veggies.

Mango Chicken Wraps

Makes 4 servings

Tortillas are lower in carbohydrates than regular bread, and chicken is a great source of protein. Choose organically raised, hormone-free poultry to avoid exposure to harmful chemicals.

Variations

Replace the mango with pineapple.

For a lower-fat version, omit the mayo or substitute low-fat soy yogurt.

¼ cup	light mayonnaise	60 mL
¼ cup	mango chutney	60 mL
4	10-inch (25 cm) multigrain tortillas	4
8 oz	cooked chicken, cut into strips	250 g
1	mango, sliced	1
¼	red onion, cut into thin rings	¼
4 cups	loosely packed mesclun mix	1 L

1. In a small bowl, combine mayonnaise and chutney.

2. Spread 2 tbsp (30 mL) of the mayonnaise mixture on each tortilla. On the bottom third of each tortilla, place one-quarter each of the chicken strips, mango slices, red onion rings and mesclun mix. Fold in the two sides, then fold the bottom of the wrap up over the filling and roll until tight.

PCOS Boost

Boost the essential fatty acid content of this recipe by adding crushed nuts.

Bulgur and Vegetable Lettuce Wraps

Here's another great sandwich alternative to help you break the bread habit. The bulgur helps fulfill the craving for starch, and the chickpeas and spices support healthy blood sugar and cholesterol levels.

Tip

People often confuse cracked wheat with bulgur. Cracked wheat is simply whole wheat grains that are crushed or cracked into smaller bits, while bulgur is wheat kernels that have been parched, steamed and dried. Bulgur is often used in Middle Eastern cooking, in dishes such as tabbouleh.

Variations

Make this recipe gluten-free by substituting cooked quinoa for the bulgur.

Use black beans or kidney beans instead of chickpeas.

For the best-quality essential fatty acids, substitute flaxseed oil for the canola oil.

Add some heat to the mixture with minced jalapeño or a few drops of hot pepper sauce.

¾ cup	bulgur	175 mL
¾ cup	warm water	175 mL
1 cup	diced tomatoes	250 mL
½ cup	cooked or canned chickpeas, drained and rinsed	125 mL
¼ cup	chopped fresh parsley	60 mL
2 tbsp	chopped green onion	30 mL
2 tbsp	chopped red onion	30 mL
1 tbsp	chopped fresh mint	15 mL
2 tbsp	canola oil	30 mL
1 tbsp	freshly squeezed lemon juice	15 mL
¼ tsp	salt	1 mL
½ tsp	freshly ground black pepper	2 mL
1	head butter lettuce, leaves separated	1

1. In a large bowl, combine bulgur and warm water. Let stand for 30 minutes, until bulgur is softened and liquid is absorbed.

2. Add tomatoes, chickpeas, parsley, green onion, red onion, mint, oil, lemon juice, salt and pepper. Stir well to combine.

3. Top each lettuce leaf with 2 tbsp (30 mL) bulgur mixture. Wrap lettuce to enclose filling.

PCOS Boost

Boost the nutrition of this recipe by substituting cooked quinoa or amaranth for the bulgur.

Salads

Citrus Fennel Slaw

Fennel offers a delicate and delicious flavor in this easy-to-prepare salad.

Tips

To get thin, even slices, use a mandoline to cut the fennel bulb.

Instead of serving on top of greens on individual plates, you can also simply pass the slaw.

Variations

Substitute toasted unsalted sunflower seeds for the pine nuts.

For the best-quality essential fatty acids, substitute flaxseed oil for the canola oil.

1	large fennel bulb	1
1/4	red onion, very thinly sliced	1/4
	Grated zest and juice of 1 lemon	
	Grated zest of 1 orange	
2 tbsp	freshly squeezed orange juice	30 mL
1 tbsp	canola oil	15 mL
Pinch	salt	Pinch
	Freshly ground black pepper	
6 cups	mesclun mix	1.5 L
3 tbsp	toasted pine nuts	45 mL

1. Remove the stalks and tough outer leaves of the fennel bulb and discard. Cut bulb in half lengthwise and trim out core. Cut bulb crosswise into very thin slices.

2. Place fennel slices and red onion in a large bowl. Stir in lemon zest, lemon juice, orange zest and orange juice. Drizzle with oil and sprinkle with salt and pepper to taste.

3. Divide mesclun mix evenly among six small plates. Mound one-sixth of the fennel slaw on each plate and garnish with pine nuts.

PCOS Boost

Boost the nutrition of this recipe by sprinkling individual servings with nutritional yeast and sprouted fenugreek. Add 1 tbsp (15 mL) prickly pear juice with the orange juice.

Spinach and Grapefruit Salad

The tart, juicy flavor of grapefruit is a delicious complement to salad greens. Make this a meal by topping the salad with canned sardines or herring, or leftover fish.

Tip

Unless your spinach comes prewashed, be sure to wash it thoroughly to remove all grit. Soak in a basin of tepid water, then rinse thoroughly under cold running water before using.

Variation

For the best-quality essential fatty acids, substitute flaxseed oil or evening primrose oil for the olive oil.

- **Blender or food processor**

2 tsp	poppy seeds	10 mL
½	red onion, thinly sliced	½
4	cloves garlic	4
3	red grapefruit	3
3 tbsp	olive oil	45 mL
2 tbsp	white wine vinegar	30 mL
2 tbsp	chopped fresh parsley	30 mL
1 tbsp	grainy mustard	15 mL
½ tsp	liquid honey	2 mL
½ tsp	salt	2 mL
¼ tsp	freshly ground black pepper	1 mL
1	bunch spinach, washed and torn into bite-size pieces	1

1. Heat a small skillet over medium heat; toast poppy seeds for 1 to 2 minutes, stirring constantly. Remove from heat. Set aside.

2. In a small bowl, cover onion with cold water; let stand for 10 minutes, then drain. In a small saucepan, cover garlic with cold water and bring to a boil; simmer for 3 minutes, then drain. Remove skins and white pith from grapefruit; cut fruit into segments, catching juice in small bowl.

3. In blender, combine garlic, oil, vinegar, parsley, mustard, honey, salt, pepper and 2 tbsp (30 mL) of the reserved grapefruit juice; blend until creamy.

4. In a large bowl, combine spinach, onion and grapefruit; toss with dressing. Garnish with reserved poppy seeds.

PCOS Boost

Boost the nutrition of this recipe by sprinkling individual servings with raw nuts and nutritional yeast. Add 1 tbsp (15 mL) prickly pear juice to the dressing.

Garden Patch Spinach Salad

Chickpeas are high in protein and provide fiber and inositol, which help regulate blood sugar levels. Spinach, carrots, peppers and tomatoes are all great sources of antioxidant vitamins and magnesium. Certainly nutritious, this salad is also delicious.

Tip

Choose organic vegetables whenever possible to reduce your chemical exposure

Variation

This salad is very versatile — vary the ingredients according to what you have on hand.

1	avocado, peeled, pitted and diced	1
4 cups	baby spinach	1 L
1 cup	grated carrot	250 mL
1 cup	julienned red bell pepper	250 mL
1 cup	grape tomatoes, halved	250 mL
1 cup	canned chickpeas, drained and rinsed	250 mL
½ cup	sunflower seeds	125 mL
¼ to ½ cup	lower-fat dressing of your choice	60 to 125 mL

1. In a large salad bowl, combine avocado, spinach, carrot, pepper, tomatoes, chickpeas and sunflower seeds. Serve with dressing on the side.

Personal Garden Herb Salad

It's important to eat at least one serving of raw foods every day, and this salad is a delicious way to do so. If you don't have any other legumes planned in the day's menu, add some canned beans to the salad.

1	tomato, cut into 8 wedges	1
1 cup	baby arugula leaves	250 mL
1/3 cup	chopped cucumber	75 mL
2 tbsp	chopped fresh oregano	30 mL
2 tbsp	chopped fresh basil	30 mL
2 tbsp	chopped fresh mint	30 mL
1 tbsp	chopped fresh chives	15 mL
1 tbsp	balsamic vinegar	15 mL
2 tsp	extra virgin olive oil	10 mL
4	kalamata olives, pitted	4
1 tbsp	crumbled feta cheese	15 mL
1/4 tsp	freshly ground black pepper	1 mL

1. In a medium bowl, combine tomato, arugula, cucumber, oregano, basil, mint and chives. Drizzle with vinegar and oil. Top with olives, cheese, pepper and salt.

Tips

To chop basil, place several leaves flat on top of each other. Roll tightly and then cut into thin strips (known as chiffonade).

It's best not to use dried herbs in this salad, as there is not enough time or moisture for them to soften and release their flavors.

Vary the amounts of the herbs to your liking.

Use all your homegrown herbs in this delightfully fresh salad, which you can double, triple or quadruple to serve up to four people.

Variation

For the best-quality essential fatty acids, substitute flaxseed oil, evening primrose oil or cod liver oil for the olive oil.

PCOS Boost

Boost the essential fatty acid content of this recipe by topping the salad with 1 tbsp (15 mL) chopped raw nuts.

Fast and Easy Greek Salad

This classic salad can be whipped up in minutes from kitchen staples.

Tip
If desired, substitute 1 tbsp (15 mL) chopped fresh basil for the dried.

Variation
For the best-quality essential fatty acids, substitute flaxseed oil for the olive oil.

2 cups	diced tomatoes	500 mL
2 cups	diced cucumbers	500 mL
1 cup	cubed feta cheese (about 8 oz/250 g)	250 mL
1/2 cup	thinly sliced onions	125 mL
1/4 cup	sliced black olives (optional)	60 mL
2 tbsp	white wine vinegar	30 mL
2 tbsp	olive oil	30 mL
1/2 tsp	minced garlic	2 mL
1/2 tsp	dried basil	2 mL
1/2 tsp	dried oregano	2 mL
	Freshly ground black pepper	

1. In a large bowl, combine tomatoes, cucumbers, cheese, onions and, if using, olives. Set aside.

2. In a small bowl or measuring cup, whisk together vinegar, oil, garlic, basil, oregano, and pepper to taste. Add to tomato mixture; toss gently to combine. Chill before serving.

> ### PCOS Boost
>
> Boost the nutrition of this recipe by sprinkling the chilled salad with nutritional yeast or topping it with fenugreek sprouts, radish sprouts or other sprouts. Increase the protein content by adding 2 tbsp (30 mL) crushed raw nuts.

Red Leaf Salad with Mango Chutney Dressing

	Makes 6 servings	

This delicious salad covers all the flavors — sweet, sour, salty, bitter and umami.

Tips

Choose organic produce whenever possible.

Much of the fat in this salad comes from the peanuts, which provide mostly unsaturated fat. If you want to reduce the total amount of fat, use 1/2 cup (125 mL) peanuts. The protein will also be reduced if you make this change.

Variations

Substitute chopped raw walnuts or pecans for the peanuts.

To keep the carbohydrate content down, substitute a pinch of stevia powder for the sugar in the dressing.

For the best-quality essential fatty acids, substitute flaxseed oil for the canola oil.

- **Blender or food processor**

8 cups	torn red leaf lettuce	2 L
1	tart apple, coarsely chopped	1
1/2 cup	sliced green onions	125 mL
1/2 cup	halved seedless red grapes	125 mL
1 cup	unsalted roasted whole peanuts	250 mL

Dressing

1 tsp	curry powder	5 mL
1/2 tsp	granulated sugar	2 mL
1/8 tsp	ground turmeric	0.5 mL
Pinch	salt	Pinch
1/4 cup	freshly squeezed lemon juice	60 mL
3 tbsp	mild or hot mango chutney	45 mL
2 tbsp	red wine vinegar	30 mL
1/4 cup	canola oil	60 mL

1. In a large bowl, combine lettuce, apple, green onions and grapes.

2. *Dressing:* In blender, combine curry powder, sugar, turmeric, salt, 1/4 cup (60 mL) water, lemon juice, chutney and vinegar; blend until smooth. With the motor running, through the feed tube, gradually add oil and process until blended.

3. Pour half the dressing over salad and toss to coat. Garnish with peanuts. Pass the remaining dressing at the table, if desired.

Snow Pea and Bell Pepper Salad

6 oz	snow peas, trimmed	175 g
4 oz	bean sprouts (or other sprouts)	125 g
1	red bell pepper, cut into strips	1
1	yellow bell pepper, cut into strips	1
1	green bell pepper, cut into strips	1
1 tbsp	sesame seeds, toasted (see tip, at left)	15 mL

Dressing

2	cloves garlic, minced	2
½ cup	orange juice	125 mL
¼ cup	olive oil	60 mL
¼ cup	red wine vinegar	60 mL

Makes 8 servings

This salad is colorful, beautiful and loaded with healthy flavonoids. Make a meal out of it by adding cooked beans or leftover or canned fish.

Tips

Toast sesame seeds in a dry skillet over medium heat, shaking occasionally, until lightly browned, about 5 minutes.

The dressing can be made ahead and stored in the refrigerator for up to 24 hours. Toss with the vegetables just before serving.

Serve with brown rice or whole wheat noodles for a delicious dinner.

1. In a small saucepan, bring 1 cup (250 mL) water to a boil. Blanch snow peas for 2 minutes or until just tender; drain and rinse under cold water. Pat dry.

2. In a large salad bowl, combine snow peas, sprouts and red, yellow and green peppers.

3. *Dressing:* In a small bowl, whisk together garlic, orange juice, oil and vinegar.

4. Pour dressing over salad and toss to coat. Sprinkle with sesame seeds.

PCOS Boost

Boost the nutrition of this recipe by topping the salad with 1 tbsp (15 mL) chopped raw nuts and 1 tsp (5 mL) nutritional yeast.

Roasted Beet, Walnut and Arugula Salad

Makes 8 servings

Beets are high in betalains and are thought to support healthy blood sugar levels, cholesterol levels and liver function. They are naturally sweet, so this salad doesn't need any sweetener beyond the orange dressing.

Tip

Toast walnuts in a dry skillet over medium heat, shaking occasionally, until lightly browned, about 5 minutes.

Variations

Substitute 4 cups (1 L) packed baby spinach for the arugula.

For the best-quality essential fatty acids, substitute flaxseed oil or borage oil for ¼ cup (60 mL) of the olive oil.

- **Preheat oven to 375°F (190°C)**

2½ lbs	fresh beets	1.25 kg
	Salt and freshly ground black pepper	
3	large oranges	3
1	shallot, finely diced	1
¼ cup	red wine vinegar	60 mL
¾ cup	extra virgin olive oil	175 mL
2	bunches (each about 5 oz/150 g) arugula, washed and trimmed	2
½ cup	toasted walnuts (see tip, at left)	125 mL

1. Wash beets and cut away tops and tails. Wrap in foil and bake in preheated oven for about 45 minutes or until just tender. Unwrap, let cool and peel under running water. Cut into chunks and season to taste with salt and pepper.

2. Meanwhile, grate the zest of 1 orange into a small bowl. Cut orange in half and squeeze juice onto the zest. Add shallot. Whisk in vinegar, then oil.

3. Peel the remaining oranges and cut into wedges.

4. Place arugula in a large salad bowl and place beets on top. Drizzle with a little orange dressing. Top with orange slices and sprinkle with walnuts. Serve the remaining dressing on the side.

PCOS Boost

Boost the nutrition of this recipe by whisking 1 tbsp (15 mL) prickly pear juice into the dressing.

Marinated Vegetable Salad

Make this salad every week or two and keep it on hand as a kitchen staple. Eat it as is, or add nuts, beans or leftover fish before serving to turn it into a meal. Top with chopped raw nuts to increase the healthy fats and add flavor and texture.

Tips

Make this salad more colorful and vary the flavor by using a variety of colored peppers and other vegetables such as snow peas or fennel, if available.

Use specialty vinegars such as tarragon, wine, champagne or balsamic to spice up the flavor of this and any salad. Try using white wine vinegar flavored with tarragon instead of the white vinegar and tarragon in this recipe.

Blanching enhances the colors of vegetables while maintaining their raw texture. To blanch vegetables, drop them into boiling water. Return to a boil and cook for 2 minutes. Drain and plunge into ice water.

Variation

For the best-quality essential fatty acids, substitute flaxseed oil for the olive oil.

½ cup	broccoli florets	125 mL
½ cup	cauliflower florets	125 mL
½ cup	sliced carrots	125 mL
½ cup	chopped green bell pepper	125 mL
½ cup	diagonally sliced celery	125 mL
½ cup	coarsely chopped English cucumber	125 mL
¼ cup	diced red or Spanish onion	60 mL
1	small tomato, cut into wedges	1

Dressing

3 tbsp	white vinegar	45 mL
1 tbsp	olive oil	15 mL
2 tsp	granulated sugar	10 mL
1½ tsp	dried oregano or tarragon	7 mL
Pinch	freshly ground black pepper	Pinch

1. In a large saucepan of boiling water, blanch broccoli, cauliflower and carrots (see tip, at left). Drain and plunge into ice water; drain again and place in medium bowl. Add green pepper, celery, cucumber and onion.

2. *Dressing:* In a small bowl or measuring cup, mix together vinegar, oil, sugar, oregano and pepper; pour over vegetables. Marinate at room temperature for 2 to 3 hours, stirring occasionally to ensure vegetables are well coated. Serve garnished with tomato wedges.

PCOS Boost

Boost the nutrition of this recipe by adding 1 tbsp (15 mL) prickly pear juice and 1 to 2 tsp (5 to 10 mL) each lecithin and brewer's yeast to the dressing. Replace the sugar with 2 tsp (10 mL) agave nectar or stevia tea, or 1 tsp (5 mL) stevia powder.

Spicy Bean Salad

Makes 6 servings

Here's another delicious way to prepare legumes. The spices in this salad bring them to life.

Tips

Smoking the dried spices — heating them in a pan without oil — intensifies their flavor.

If desired, substitute 1 cup (250 mL) dried beans, cooked and drained, for the canned version.

Variation

For the best-quality essential fatty acids, substitute flaxseed oil for the olive oil.

2 tsp	ground cumin	10 mL
1 tsp	curry powder	5 mL
1	can (14 oz/398 mL) kidney beans, drained and rinsed	1
½	Spanish or red onion, diced	½
2	tomatoes, chopped	2
2	stalks celery, chopped	2
2	green onions, sliced	2
2 tbsp	freshly squeezed lime juice	30 mL
1 tbsp	olive oil	15 mL
¼ cup	chopped fresh cilantro	60 mL

1. In a dry skillet, heat cumin and curry powder over high heat until fragrant. Remove from heat and set aside.

2. In a large bowl, combine vegetables.

3. Mix lime juice and olive oil with roasted spices; pour over bean mixture. Stir in cilantro. Cover and chill thoroughly.

PCOS Boost

Boost the chromium content of this recipe by adding 1 to 2 tsp (5 to 10 mL) brewer's yeast to the spices.

Colorful Bean and Corn Salad

Corn produces a high glycemic load, but when it's combined with beans and other vegetables, the fiber blunts the spike in glucose levels. Use fresh organic corn, cooked and cut from the cob, when available.

Tip

If you're in a hurry, give the dressing a pass and add ½ tsp (2 mL) cumin to ¼ cup (60 mL) bottled oil-and-vinegar salad dressing.

Salad

1	can (19 oz/540 mL) black beans, drained and rinsed (about 2 cups/ 500 mL)	1
1	can (12 oz/341 mL) corn kernels, drained	1
1 cup	chopped tomatoes	250 mL
½ cup	chopped green or red bell pepper	125 mL
½ cup	chopped red onion	125 mL
¼ cup	chopped fresh parsley	60 mL

Dressing

2 tbsp	red wine vinegar or balsamic vinegar	30 mL
1 tbsp	olive oil	15 mL
½ tsp	ground cumin	2 mL
½ tsp	minced garlic	2 mL
½ tsp	hot pepper sauce (optional)	2 mL
¼ tsp	salt	1 mL
	Freshly ground black pepper	

1. *Salad:* In a large bowl, combine beans, corn, tomatoes, pepper, onion and parsley. Set aside.

2. *Dressing:* In a small bowl or measuring cup, whisk together vinegar, oil, cumin, garlic, hot pepper sauce, if using, salt and pepper to taste. Blend well. Pour over salad.

PCOS Boost

Boost the chromium content of this recipe by adding 1 tsp (5 mL) each brewer's yeast and lecithin to the dressing.

Mediterranean Lentil and Rice Salad

Makes 10 servings

Brown rice is higher in fiber and lower on the glycemic index than white rice. You can rely on the sweetness of the peppers and apricots to carry the flavor and omit the honey from the dressing.

Tips

For 3 cups (750 mL) cooked brown rice, cook 1 cup (250 mL) rice with 2 cups (500 mL) water.

If you serve this as a main course instead of as a side salad, it serves 6.

This salad keeps well for up to 1 week in the refrigerator.

Variation

To lower the glycemic load of this salad, use agave nectar instead of honey, or try stevia powder, which improves insulin resistance in PCOS.

2	roasted red bell peppers, patted dry and julienned	2
1	can (19 oz/540 mL) lentils, drained and rinsed (about 2 cups/500 mL)	1
3 cups	cooked brown rice	750 mL
1 cup	chopped fresh Italian (flat-leaf) parsley	250 mL
½ cup	thinly sliced green onions	125 mL
¼ cup	slivered dried apricots	60 mL

Dressing

¼ cup	olive oil	60 mL
2 tbsp	freshly squeezed lemon juice	30 mL
2 tbsp	balsamic vinegar	30 mL
1 tsp	liquid honey	5 mL
1 tsp	ground cumin	5 mL
½ tsp	ground coriander	2 mL
	Salt and freshly ground black pepper	

1. In a large bowl, combine red peppers, lentils, rice, parsley, green onions and apricots.

2. *Dressing:* In a small bowl, whisk together olive oil, lemon juice, vinegar, honey, cumin, coriander and salt and pepper to taste.

3. Pour dressing over salad and toss to coat.

PCOS Boost

Boost the nutrition of this recipe by substituting cooked quinoa or amaranth for the rice.

Bulgur Salad with Broccoli, Radishes and Celery

<table>
<tr><td>Makes 8 servings</td></tr>
</table>

Bulgur is lower on the glycemic index than bread or rolls, but is equally satisfying. The texture is delightfully chewy.

Tip

Cooking the vinegar, mustard and garlic along with the broth intensifies the flavor of the cooked bulgur.

Variations

Use freshly squeezed lemon juice instead of vinegar.

Add ½ cup (125 mL) mixed chopped fresh herbs, such as basil, oregano, tarragon and thyme.

For added protein and fiber, add 1 cup (250 mL) cooked chickpeas, lentils or black beans.

- Steamer basket

1½ cups	broccoli florets	375 mL
1	clove garlic, minced	1
¾ cup	reduced-sodium chicken broth	175 mL
3 tbsp	red wine vinegar	45 mL
1½ tsp	Dijon mustard	7 mL
1 cup	bulgur	250 mL
⅓ cup	chopped radishes	75 mL
⅓ cup	chopped celery	75 mL
⅓ cup	chopped red bell pepper	75 mL
¼ cup	chopped green onions	60 mL
1½ tbsp	extra virgin olive oil	22 mL
½ tsp	freshly ground black pepper	2 mL
¼ tsp	salt	1 mL

1. In a large pot fitted with a steamer basket, steam broccoli for 4 to 5 minutes or until tender-crisp. Drain and set aside.

2. In a medium saucepan, combine garlic, broth, vinegar and mustard; bring to a boil over high heat. Remove from heat and stir in bulgur. Cover and let stand for 15 minutes. Fluff with a fork.

3. Add broccoli, radishes, celery, red pepper and green onions to bulgur mixture and stir to combine. Gently stir in oil, pepper and salt.

PCOS Boost

Boost the nutrition of this recipe by adding 1 tbsp (15 mL) lecithin and 1 tsp (5 mL) brewer's yeast with the bulgur. Top each serving with 1 tbsp (15 mL) chopped raw nuts.

Vegetable Quinoa Salad

Quinoa is higher in protein than most grains and offers a refreshing alternative to wheat, rice or oats. Give it a try.

Tips

If you are not a fan of the strong flavors of hot pepper flakes and/or lavender, leave them out. You could also substitute your favorite homemade or store-bought dressing; ¼ cup (60 mL) is required to coat the salad. Remember, you do not want it soaked in dressing, just enough to enhance the natural flavors.

Only lavender that has been grown specifically for food use should be used in cooking. Avoid lavender sold for decoration or potpourri, as it may have been treated to preserve the color.

This salad is best served fresh, but it will keep for up to 2 days in the refrigerator.

1 cup	quinoa, well rinsed and drained	250 mL
2 cups	cold water	500 mL
2	tomatoes, chopped	2
2	large sprigs Italian (flat-leaf) parsley (leaves only), chopped	2
¼	English cucumber, chopped	¼
⅓ cup	chopped red, green, yellow or mixed bell peppers	75 mL

Vinaigrette

3 tbsp	extra virgin olive oil	45 mL
2 tbsp	freshly squeezed lemon juice	30 mL
1½ tsp	hot pepper flakes (optional)	7 mL
½ tsp	salt	2 mL
½ tsp	freshly ground black pepper	2 mL
½ tsp	dried lavender flowers (optional)	2 mL

1. In a medium saucepan, over medium heat, bring quinoa and water to a boil. Reduce heat and boil gently for 10 to 15 minutes or until the white germ separates from the seed. Cover, remove from heat and let stand for 5 minutes. Remove lid, let cool and fluff with a fork.

2. Meanwhile, in a large bowl, combine tomatoes, parsley, cucumber and bell peppers. Stir in cooled quinoa.

3. *Vinaigrette:* In a small bowl, whisk together olive oil, lemon juice, hot pepper flakes (if using), salt, pepper and lavender (if using).

4. Pour vinaigrette over salad and toss to coat.

PCOS Boost

Boost the nutrition of this recipe by topping the salad with chopped raw nuts, sprouted fenugreek and nutritional yeast.

Chicken and Bean Salad

This high-protein salad could be a meal in itself, or you can eat some with dinner and take the leftovers to work the next day for a nutritious and delicious lunch.

Tips

For a change, try substituting black beans or chickpeas for the kidney beans.

If desired, use 1 cup (250 mL) dried beans, soaked, cooked, drained and rinsed, instead of the canned version.

This recipe is a great way to use up leftover chicken, but you can also use a small cooked chicken from your grocery store. Pick up a bag of ready-to-use salad greens and you're almost ready for supper.

Choose organic chicken to avoid exposure to hormones and chemicals.

For the best-quality essential fatty acids, use flaxseed oil or borage oil.

1	can (14 oz/398 mL) kidney beans, drained and rinsed	1
1 cup	corn kernels, canned or frozen	250 mL
1 cup	cubed cooked chicken	250 mL
¾ cup	diced red bell peppers	175 mL
2	green onions, chopped	2
¼ cup	red wine vinegar	60 mL
2 tbsp	vegetable oil	30 mL
½ tsp	minced garlic	2 mL
¼ tsp	salt	1 mL
¼ tsp	freshly ground black pepper	1 mL
¼ to ½ tsp	hot pepper sauce (optional)	1 to 2 mL

1. In a medium bowl, combine beans, corn, chicken, peppers, onions, vinegar, oil, garlic, salt, pepper and, if using, hot pepper sauce. Toss gently until combined. Chill before serving.

Grilled Salmon, Mango and Raspberry Spinach Salad

Featuring grilled salmon and tossed in a raspberry vinaigrette, this salad is a meal in and of itself, and is pleasing to the eye and the palate. Salmon is high in healthy fats and is a good source of protein.

Tip

To avoid cross-contamination, use separate brushes to baste the onions and salmon.

Variation

Use a combination of blueberries, blackberries and raspberries in the salad.

- Preheat barbecue grill to medium
- Blender or food processor
- Two 12-inch (30 cm) bamboo skewers, soaked

Raspberry Vinaigrette

⅔ cup	fresh or frozen raspberries (thawed and drained if frozen)	150 mL
3 tbsp	balsamic vinegar	45 mL
1 tbsp	liquid honey	15 mL
2 tbsp	water	30 mL
½ tsp	Dijon mustard	2 mL
¼ tsp	freshly ground black pepper	1 mL
2 tbsp	canola or olive oil	30 mL
1 tbsp	finely chopped shallots	15 mL

Salad

1	red onion, cut into 8 wedges	1
4	salmon steaks (about 1 lb/500 g total)	4
6 cups	lightly packed baby spinach	1.5 L
1	ripe mango, thinly sliced	1
1 cup	fresh raspberries	250 mL

1. *Vinaigrette:* Purée raspberries in blender. Press through a sieve to remove seeds.

2. In a small bowl, whisk together puréed raspberries, vinegar, honey, 2 tbsp (30 mL) water, mustard and pepper. Gradually whisk in oil until blended. Stir in shallots. Divide vinaigrette in half. Set half aside for end and use half for grilling.

3. *Salad:* Thread 4 onion wedges onto each skewer and brush with some of the vinaigrette for grilling. Brush salmon on both sides with vinaigrette. Place skewers and salmon on preheated grill, close lid and grill, basting frequently with vinaigrette and turning once, for 10 minutes or until fish is opaque and flakes easily when tested with a fork.

4. Remove onions from skewers and place in a salad bowl. Add spinach, mango, raspberries and reserved vinaigrette; toss to coat. Divide salad among four plates and top each with grilled salmon.

Black-Eyed Pea Salad with Cajun Chicken

Black-eyed peas are said to bring good luck! It will certainly be your good luck to eat this salad, which is both flavorful and nutritious.

Tips

Both black-eyed peas and black beans, popular in Southern-style recipes, are available canned in many supermarkets, as are several brands of Cajun seasoning.

If desired, replace the canned legumes with 1 cup (250 mL) dried black-eyed peas or black beans, soaked, cooked, drained and rinsed.

Instead of watercress, use 2 cups (500 mL) shredded spinach or romaine lettuce, if desired.

1	can (14 oz/398 mL) black-eyed peas or black beans	1
3	green onions, chopped	3
1	small bunch watercress	1
1	carrot, grated	1
1	apple (unpeeled), cubed	1
$\frac{2}{3}$ cup	bottled no-fat vinaigrette	150 mL
8 oz	boneless skinless chicken breasts	250 g
1 tsp	olive oil	5 mL
1 to 2 tsp	Cajun seasoning	5 to 10 mL
	Russian rye bread (optional)	

1. Drain and rinse peas. In a bowl, combine peas, green onions, watercress, carrot and apple; toss with dressing. Cover and chill for 30 minutes.

2. Slice chicken breasts lengthwise into 8 thin strips. Coat with oil and Cajun seasoning. In a hot skillet, cook chicken until browned and no longer pink inside, about 5 minutes. Serve with salad and bread, if desired.

PCOS Boost

Boost the chromium and *D-chiro-inositol* content of this recipe by adding 2 tsp (10 mL) lecithin and $\frac{1}{2}$ tsp (2 mL) brewer's yeast with the dressing.

Main Dishes

Chickpea Hot Pot

2 tsp	olive oil	10 mL
½ cup	chopped onions	125 mL
1 tbsp	curry paste	15 mL
2	cans (each 28 oz/796 mL) diced plum tomatoes, with juice	2
1	can (19 oz/540 mL) chickpeas, drained and rinsed (about 2 cups/500 mL)	1
1 cup	diced sweet potatoes	250 mL
1 tbsp	granulated sugar	15 mL
1 tsp	minced garlic	5 mL
1 cup	cubed firm tofu	250 mL
2 cups	bok choy, cut into strips	500 mL
2 cups	broccoli florets	500 mL
½ tsp	freshly ground black pepper	2 mL

Makes 6 servings

This chickpea-based dinner demonstrates the versatility of legumes. Make it even more appealing by topping each bowl with sesame seeds and sprouts.

Tips

Curry paste is available in Asian markets or the specialty section of some supermarkets.

You can substitute black beans or red kidney beans for the chickpeas. Add more curry paste if you like spice.

Variation

Omit the sugar, or substitute 2 tsp (10 mL) agave nectar or ½ tsp (2 mL) stevia powder.

1. In a saucepan, heat oil over medium-high heat. Add onions and cook until softened. Stir in curry paste. Add tomatoes, chickpeas, sweet potatoes, sugar and garlic; bring to a boil. Reduce heat and simmer, covered, until sweet potatoes are tender.

2. Stir in tofu, bok choy, broccoli and pepper. Cook, uncovered, for 2 minutes or until broccoli is tender-crisp. Adjust seasoning to taste.

PCOS Boost

Boost the chromium and *D-chiro-inositol* content of this recipe by adding 2 tbsp (30 mL) lecithin and 2 tsp (10 mL) each brewer's yeast and nutritional yeast. If you like garlic, use double or even triple the amount to increase the benefit to your blood sugar and cholesterol levels.

Falafels

Falafels are a traditional Middle Eastern food typically served in pitas, but the patties are also great crumbled into salads or on top of soups. The chickpeas and spices support healthy blood sugar and cholesterol.

Tips

Tahini is available in health food stores and the specialty foods section of many supermarkets.

The seasonings may be increased to suit your taste.

Extra bread crumbs will give a drier patty.

- **Food processor or blender**

1	can (19 oz/540 mL) chickpeas, drained (reserve liquid) and rinsed (about 2 cups/500 mL)	1
2	large cloves garlic	2
1	small onion, chopped	1
½ cup	packed parsley leaves	125 mL
⅓ cup	tahini (sesame seed paste)	75 mL
2 tbsp	freshly squeezed lemon juice	30 mL
1 tbsp	ground cumin	15 mL
1 tsp	ground coriander	5 mL
1 tsp	ground turmeric	5 mL
½ tsp	salt	2 mL
¼ tsp	freshly ground black pepper	1 mL
¼ cup	dry bread crumbs	60 mL
1 tbsp	vegetable oil	15 mL
4	whole wheat pita breads	4
	Shredded lettuce, chopped tomatoes, diced cucumber, alfalfa sprouts, plain yogurt	

1. In food processor, process chickpeas, 2 tbsp (30 mL) of the reserved liquid, garlic, onion, parsley, tahini, lemon juice and seasonings; process until almost smooth. Stir in bread crumbs; shape into 8 patties.

2. In a large nonstick skillet over medium-high heat, heat oil. Add patties; cook for 2 to 3 minutes per side or until lightly browned. Cut pita breads in half; serve each patty in pocket of half a pita bread; garnish as desired.

PCOS Boost

Boost the nutrition of this recipe by adding 1 tbsp (15 mL) lecithin and 1 tsp (5 mL) brewer's yeast with the seasonings. To increase the essential fatty acid content, sprinkle each serving with 1½ tsp (7 mL) each sesame seeds and ground flax seeds (flaxseed meal).

Mexican Pie

Here's yet another delicious way to eat legumes. Use a heat-stable oil, such as walnut oil, and shop at a health food store for a good-quality coarse organic cornmeal.

Tips

To turn up the heat, add a finely chopped jalapeño pepper along with the tomatoes.

If desired, use 1 cup (250 mL) dried kidney beans, soaked, cooked and drained, instead of the canned.

The beans, cornmeal, cheese, milk and eggs combine to provide high-quality protein in the absence of meat. To add extra fiber, serve with a spinach salad and a multigrain roll.

Variations

To reduce the fat content of this recipe, substitute soy milk for the cow's milk.

Substitute chopped organic ripe fresh tomatoes for canned tomatoes, which can contain bisphenols in the plasticized can lining.

- Preheat oven to 350°F (180°C)
- 13- by 9-inch (33 by 23 cm) baking dish

1	onion, chopped	1
1 tbsp	vegetable oil	15 mL
1	can (19 oz/540 mL) tomatoes, coarsely chopped	1
1	can (14 oz/398 mL) kidney beans, drained and rinsed	1
1	can (12 oz/341 mL) whole kernel corn	1
1 tbsp	chili powder	15 mL
¾ cup	cornmeal	175 mL
1 cup	2% milk	250 mL
2	eggs	2
1½ cups	shredded cheese (sharp/old Cheddar, Swiss, mozzarella or a combination)	375 mL

1. In a large skillet over medium-high heat, cook onion in oil until transparent. Add tomatoes, kidney beans, corn and chili powder to skillet. Cook over low heat, uncovered, for about 1 hour or until slightly thickened, stirring occasionally. Pour mixture into baking dish. Sprinkle cornmeal evenly over surface.

2. In a bowl, beat together milk and eggs; pour evenly over cornmeal. Sprinkle with cheese. Bake in preheated oven for 50 to 55 minutes. Cut into squares to serve.

PCOS Boost

Boost the nutrition of this recipe by sprinkling individual servings with ground flax seeds (flaxseed meal), nutritional yeast and sprouts.

Garden Path Burgers

These vegetarian burgers have it all: lentils, quinoa, chickpeas and rolled oats. For the healthiest meal, omit the bun and eat one plain, served with a topping of chopped tomatoes, grated carrots and minced onions.

Tip

Be sure to use extra-firm tofu in this recipe as other textures are not firm enough to be shredded.

Variations

Reduce the bread crumbs to 1 cup (250 mL) and add 2 cups (500 mL) nut flour and ground flax seeds (flaxseed meal).

For a spicier version, add finely chopped hot pepper, such as jalapeño or banana pepper, along with the bell peppers.

- Preheat oven to 375°F (190°C)
- Baking sheet

1/4 cup	dried lentils	60 mL
1/4 cup	quinoa	60 mL
3 cups	fine dry bread crumbs	750 mL
1/4 cup	quick-cooking rolled oats	60 mL
1/4 cup	chopped walnuts	60 mL
1 cup	coarsely chopped canned chickpeas, drained and rinsed	250 mL
2/3 cup	finely chopped carrot	150 mL
2/3 cup	finely chopped celery	150 mL
2/3 cup	finely chopped Spanish onion	150 mL
1/2 cup	finely chopped red bell pepper	125 mL
1/2 cup	finely chopped green bell pepper	125 mL
1/2 cup	shredded extra-firm tofu	125 mL
1/4 cup	sliced green onions	60 mL
1/4 cup	toasted pumpkin seeds	60 mL
1 tbsp	coarsely cracked black pepper	15 mL
12	onion or vegetable Kaiser buns, split and toasted	12

Toppings

Light mayonnaise, bean sprouts, sliced tomato, chopped fresh cilantro, shredded lettuce

1. In a medium saucepan, combine lentils, quinoa and 1 1/2 cups (375 mL) water; bring to a boil. Reduce heat and simmer for 10 minutes; drain.

2. In a large bowl, mix together lentil mixture, bread crumbs, rolled oats, walnuts, chickpeas, carrot, celery, onion, red and green peppers, tofu, green onions, pumpkin seeds and pepper. Using 1 cup (250 mL) for each, form into 1/2-inch (1 cm) thick patties about 3 inches (8 cm) in diameter.

3. Bake on baking sheet in preheated oven for about 20 minutes or until hot and golden brown. Serve on buns with favorite toppings.

Stir-Fried Vegetables with Tofu

This vegetable-packed dish is naturally high in nutrients and fiber, and tofu is a good source of protein. To lower the glycemic load, substitute arrowroot powder for the cornstarch.

Tip

Tofu is best stored in water in a covered container in the refrigerator. Change the water daily to keep tofu fresh for 1 week.

2 tbsp	vegetable oil	30 mL
1	large onion, cut into wedges	1
3	carrots, sliced diagonally	3
3	celery stalks, sliced diagonally	3
1/4	small cabbage, sliced thinly	1/4
1 cup	snow peas, trimmed	250 mL
1 cup	sliced mushrooms	250 mL
1 cup	firm tofu, cubed	250 mL
1/2 cup	chicken broth	125 mL
1 tbsp	cornstarch	15 mL
1 tsp	finely chopped gingerroot (or 1/2 tsp/2 mL ground ginger)	5 mL
1/4 tsp	freshly ground black pepper	1 mL

1. In a wok or large heavy skillet, heat oil over high heat. When oil is very hot, add onion, carrot and celery; cover and steam for 5 minutes. Add cabbage, snow peas, mushrooms and tofu; steam, covered, for 5 minutes longer.

2. Mix together chicken broth, cornstarch, ginger and pepper; pour over vegetable mixture. Stir-fry for 1 minute or until sauce thickens. Serve over hot rice.

PCOS Boost

Boost the essential fatty acid content of this recipe by sprinkling individual servings with sesame seeds and ground flax seeds (flaxseed meal).

Poached Fish Jardinière

Fish offers good-quality fats, especially omega-3 fatty acids, and is a good source of protein, so eat it several times a week. Serve with cooked vegetables and a raw salad.

Tips

When using bay leaves in cooking, keep them whole or break into large pieces so that they can be easily removed before serving.

If desired, use fresh tarragon and chervil in this recipe. Double or triple the quantity, depending on your taste, and add some finely chopped leaves as a garnish.

Chervil, a herb often used in French cuisine, resembles parsley with a licorice taste. If you don't have chervil in your cupboard, add 2 tbsp (30 mL) fresh parsley to the sauce.

- Preheat oven to 425°F (220°C)
- Large, shallow baking dish

1	small onion, chopped	1
6 to 8	bay leaves	6 to 8
6 to 8	portions (each about 4 oz/125 g) fresh or frozen halibut or haddock	6 to 8
6 to 8	thin slices lemon	6 to 8
1 cup	dry white wine	250 mL
½ cup	water	125 mL
Sauce		
4	large tomatoes, chopped	4
2	cloves garlic, minced	2
¼ cup	plain yogurt	60 mL
2 tbsp	olive oil	30 mL
2 tbsp	chopped fresh parsley	30 mL
1 tbsp	Dijon mustard	15 mL
2 tsp	dried chervil	10 mL
2 tsp	dried tarragon	10 mL
1 tsp	Worcestershire sauce	5 mL
¼ tsp	salt	1 mL
	Freshly ground black pepper	

1. Spread onion on bottom of dish. Place bay leaves in dish; top each with piece of fish and lemon slice. Pour wine and water over top. Cover and chill for at least 1 hour.

2. *Sauce:* In a saucepan, combine tomatoes, garlic, yogurt, oil, parsley, mustard, chervil, tarragon, Worcestershire sauce, salt and pepper to taste; cook over low heat for 10 to 15 minutes to blend flavors. (Do not boil.)

3. Bake fish in preheated oven for 10 to 15 minutes or until fish flakes easily when tested with fork. Remove fish from liquid and arrange on plates, adding some liquid to sauce for desired consistency if necessary. Pour sauce over fish.

PCOS Boost

Boost the nutrition of this recipe by adding 1 tbsp (15 mL) prickly pear juice to the sauce. Use double the amount of garlic if you like the flavor.

Asian Fish Fillets

Delicious with ginger and cilantro, fish is a great source of protein and provides healthy fats.

Tips

Don't confuse cilantro with parsley. They look similar but they are different. Cilantro is the parsley-like leaf on the coriander plant. Cilantro leaves are more tender than parsley and have a zesty, almost bitter, flavor that lingers on the tongue.

Look for reduced-sodium soy sauce at health food stores and well-stocked supermarkets.

4	green onions, diagonally sliced	4
2	cloves garlic, minced	2
1 tbsp	canola oil	15 mL
4	fish fillets (turbot, cod, haddock or halibut)	4
1 tbsp	finely chopped gingerroot	15 mL
½ cup	dry sherry	125 mL
2 tbsp	soy sauce	30 mL
¼ cup	coarsely chopped fresh cilantro	60 mL

1. In a heavy skillet over high heat, cook green onions and garlic in hot oil for about 2 minutes. Remove onion mixture and add fish to skillet.

2. Combine onion mixture, gingerroot, sherry and soy sauce; pour over fish. Sprinkle with cilantro. Cook, covered, over medium heat for about 5 minutes or until fish flakes easily when tested with fork. Transfer fillets to preheated platter. Cook sauce over high heat until reduced and slightly thickened. Pour sauce over fish and serve.

PCOS Boost

Boost the essential fatty acid content of this recipe by garnishing individual servings with chopped raw nuts.

Tandoori Haddock

Here's another delectable fish option to add to the weekly rotation. Serve with a side salad and steamed broccoli. Cook an extra fillet to add to a breakfast tray or a lunch salad.

Tip

Most supermarkets now carry tandoori paste. You can usually find it in the ethnic food aisle where Indian and Asian sauces are displayed.

Variation

This works well with most firm white fish fillets or steaks, such as halibut or orange roughy. We have even tested it with salmon, and it works great! Adjust the broiling time depending on the thickness of the fish.

- **Rimmed baking sheet, lightly greased**

¼ cup	tandoori paste (see tip, at left)	60 mL
¼ cup	low-fat plain yogurt	60 mL
1 tbsp	freshly squeezed lemon juice	15 mL
4	haddock fillets (about 14 oz/420 g total)	4

1. In a shallow dish, combine tandoori paste, yogurt and lemon juice. Add fish, turning to coat evenly. Cover and refrigerate for 20 to 30 minutes. Meanwhile, preheat broiler, with rack set 4 inches (10 cm) from the top.

2. Place fish on baking sheet and broil for 10 minutes or until fish is opaque and flakes easily with a fork and the top is lightly browned.

PCOS Boost

Boost the nutrition of this recipe by adding several whole garlic cloves to the baking sheet with the fish. Garlic benefits your blood sugar and cholesterol levels.

Pan-Seared Mahi Mahi with Papaya Mint Relish

A delicious relish adds pizzazz to pan-seared fish. Aim to eat fish at least two or three times a week to benefit from its high-quality essential fatty acids and easy-to-digest protein. Serve with a cooked vegetable, such as mashed squash, steamed Brussels sprouts or roasted veggies.

Tips

Substitute sea bass or halibut if mahi mahi is not available.

If papaya is not in season, use fresh or canned pineapple or mango instead.

Papaya Mint Relish

1½ cups	diced peeled papaya (1 large)	375 mL
⅓ cup	finely diced shallots or green onions	75 mL
3 tbsp	finely chopped fresh mint	45 mL
2 tbsp	freshly squeezed lime juice	30 mL
Pinch	salt	Pinch
Pinch	freshly ground black pepper	Pinch
Pinch	granulated sugar	Pinch

Fish

2 tbsp	all-purpose flour	30 mL
Pinch	salt	Pinch
Pinch	black pepper	Pinch
4	mahi mahi fillets (each about 3 oz/90 g)	4
1 tbsp	extra virgin olive oil	15 mL

1. *Relish:* In a small bowl, mix papaya, shallots, mint, lime juice, salt, pepper and sugar; set aside.

2. *Fish:* Mix together flour, salt and pepper; dip fish fillets into flour to coat both sides. In a nonstick pan, heat oil over medium-high heat; cook fish for 1½ to 3 minutes per side or until fish flakes easily when tested with a fork. Serve topped with relish.

PCOS Boost

Boost the nutrition of this recipe by adding 1 to 2 tbsp (15 to 30 mL) prickly pear juice and 1 tbsp (15 mL) lecithin to the relish.

Salmon Medallions with Two Purées

Makes 6 servings

Two delicious purées add color and variety to a healthy meal. Serve with veggies.

Tips

Sauces do not need to be high in fat. These vegetable purées add elegance, color, flavor and nutrients to this dish, but no fat. Enjoy this salmon with rice and a side salad for a special lunch.

When puréeing a small quantity of food, such as these two sauces, use an immersion blender for convenience.

- **Food processor or blender**

Cherry Tomato Purée

10	cherry tomatoes	10
1 tbsp	sliced green onion	15 mL
1½ tsp	soy sauce	7 mL
¼ tsp	Worcestershire sauce	1 mL
¼ tsp	salt	1 mL

Beet Purée

¾ cup	chopped cooked beets	175 mL
2 tbsp	water	30 mL
1 tbsp	chopped onion	15 mL
1 tbsp	red wine vinegar	15 mL
¼ tsp	salt	1 mL

Fish

1¼ lbs	salmon fillets	625 g
	Freshly ground black pepper	
1 tbsp	vegetable oil	15 mL
	Chopped fresh chives	

1. *Cherry Tomato Purée:* In food processor, process tomatoes, green onion, soy sauce, Worcestershire sauce and salt until smooth. Pour into a small bowl and chill.

2. *Beet Purée:* In clean food processor, process beets, water, onion, vinegar and salt until smooth. Pour into a small bowl and chill.

3. *Fish:* Place salmon in freezer for 30 minutes to aid slicing. Slice diagonally into 6 thin medallions. Sprinkle with pepper to taste. In a skillet, heat oil over medium-high heat; quickly cook salmon, about 1 minute per side.

4. To serve, place salmon on plate; spoon purées around salmon. Garnish with chives.

Asian Salmon

In this recipe, hoisin sauce and spice permeate the fish, giving it a rich, complex flavor. Serve with raw and cooked vegetables to round out the meal.

Tips

Hoisin sauce, an extremely flavorful sauce made with soybeans, garlic and other spices, contains a lot of sodium, so use it sparingly.

You can substitute red or white wine vinegar if you don't have rice vinegar.

Use any leftover salmon to make salmon cakes or salmon salad.

This marinade also works well for chicken, pork, shrimp or scallops and makes a great stir-fry sauce for noodle or rice dishes.

Variation

Omit the honey or substitute ¼ tsp (1 mL) stevia powder.

- Preheat oven to 375°F (190°C)
- Rimmed baking sheet, lined with foil, then parchment paper

1	garlic clove, finely minced	1
2 tsp	finely minced gingerroot	10 mL
Pinch	hot pepper flakes	Pinch
¼ cup	hoisin sauce	60 mL
1 tbsp	rice vinegar	15 mL
1 tbsp	liquid honey	15 mL
2 tsp	reduced-sodium soy sauce	10 mL
1 tsp	sesame oil	5 mL
4	pieces skinless salmon fillet (about 1 lb/500 g total)	4

1. In a small bowl, stir together garlic, ginger, hot pepper flakes, hoisin sauce, vinegar, honey, soy sauce and oil. Transfer all but 2 tbsp (30 mL) marinade to a sealable plastic bag. Add salmon fillets and distribute marinade to coat salmon. Seal bag and let stand at room temperature for 10 minutes or refrigerate for up to 2 hours.

2. Remove salmon from marinade and place on prepared baking sheet. Discard marinade from bag.

3. Bake in preheated oven, basting once with the reserved marinade, for 10 to 12 minutes or until fish is opaque and flakes easily when tested with a fork.

PCOS Boost

Boost the nutrition of this recipe by adding 1 tbsp (15 mL) prickly pear juice and 1 tbsp (15 mL) lecithin to the marinade.

Pepper-Crusted Rainbow Trout

This simple recipe can be prepared in a matter of minutes. Make an extra fillet or two to eat for breakfast or to add to a lunch salad.

Tips

This seems like a lot of pepper, but it yields a delicious, spicy flavor.

Keep your kitchen fan on to quickly remove any excess smoke that may be generated from searing the fish at a high heat.

Variation

Use salmon or Arctic char instead of trout and increase the cooking time in step 3 as necessary.

¼ cup	coarsely ground black pepper	60 mL
¼ tsp	coarse sea salt	1 mL
4	rainbow trout fillets (about 1 lb/500 g total)	4
1 tbsp	canola oil	15 mL
1 cup	dry white wine	250 mL
¼ cup	freshly squeezed lemon juice	60 mL

1. In a large, shallow dish, combine pepper and salt; spread out over bottom of dish. Firmly press trout fillets, flesh side down, into pepper mixture, coating flesh completely (do not coat the skin side). Shake off excess and set aside on a clean plate. Discard any excess pepper mixture.

2. In a large skillet, heat oil over medium-high heat until hot but not smoking. In batches as necessary, place fillets, flesh side down, in skillet. Cover and cook for 1 to 2 minutes or until fish is brown and crispy. Transfer fish to a plate. Repeat with the remaining fillets.

3. Return trout to pan, flesh side up. Reduce heat to medium-low and add wine and lemon juice to the skillet. Cover and cook for 8 to 10 minutes or until fish is opaque and flakes easily when tested with a fork. If pan begins to dry out, add 1 to 2 tbsp (15 to 30 mL) water.

PCOS Boost

Boost the nutrition of this recipe by adding 1 tbsp (15 mL) lecithin and 1 tsp (5 mL) brewer's yeast with the lemon juice.

Grilled Chicken with Stir-Fried Vegetables

This makes a great dinner for a single person or a couple, with enough left over to pack into containers for lunches.

Tips

Choose organic chicken to avoid exposure to hormones and chemicals.

To prevent food from sticking when stir-frying, heat the pan before adding the oil. Tip the pan to distribute the oil evenly across the bottom and around the sides. Return the pan to the element. When the oil is just smoking, begin to fry, using large spatulas to stir the vegetables.

- Preheat barbecue or broiler

4	boneless skinless chicken breasts (each about 3 oz/90 g)	4
1	lime	1
1 tsp	soy sauce	5 mL
4	stalks celery	4
1	red bell pepper	1
1	green bell pepper	1
1	large onion	1
1	carrot	1
1½ tsp	ground cumin	7 mL
1½ tsp	chili powder	7 mL
1 tsp	ground lemon pepper	5 mL
½ cup	chicken broth	125 mL

1. Using meat mallet, pound chicken between plastic wrap to ⅜-inch (9 mm) thickness. Place chicken in glass dish; squeeze lime juice over all. Coat with soy sauce. Set aside.

2. Cut celery on angle ⅛ inch (3 mm) thick and 2 inches (5 cm) long. Cut red and green peppers and onion into long thin strips. Using peeler, peel carrot into long thin strips. Combine vegetables with cumin, chili powder and lemon pepper. Set aside.

3. Broil or barbecue chicken until no longer pink, 4 to 5 minutes per side.

4. Meanwhile, in a large nonstick skillet sprayed with nonstick cooking spray, cook vegetables, stirring, until hot. Stir in chicken broth; cook until vegetables are tender, about 8 minutes. Serve over chicken.

PCOS Boost

Boost the essential fatty acid content of this recipe by sprinkling individual servings with ground flax seeds (flaxseed meal) and chopped raw walnuts or cashews.

Thai Turkey Stir-Fry

This flavorful, easy-to-prepare dinner is high in protein and full of nutrient-dense veggies. Serve with brown rice or quinoa for a meal with a low glycemic load.

Tips

Use a heat-stable oil, such as walnut oil.

Choose organic turkey to avoid exposure to hormones and chemicals.

Finish the meal with tropical fruits, such as mango, pineapple and papaya.

1 tbsp	vegetable oil	15 mL
2	cloves garlic, finely chopped	2
1	2-inch (5 cm) piece gingerroot, grated	1
1 lb	boneless skinless turkey breast, cut into strips	500 g
1	head bok choy (about 1 lb/500 g), chopped	1
1	red bell pepper, julienned	1
½ cup	light coconut milk	125 mL
1 tsp	grated lime zest	5 mL
2 tbsp	freshly squeezed lime juice	30 mL
1 tbsp	reduced-sodium soy sauce	15 mL
1 tsp	red curry paste	5 mL
	Salt and freshly ground black pepper	
2 tsp	chopped fresh cilantro	10 mL

1. Heat a wok or large skillet over medium-high heat. Add oil and swirl to coat wok. Sauté garlic, ginger and turkey for about 10 minutes or until turkey is lightly browned on the outside and no longer pink inside. Add bok choy and red pepper; sauté for 4 minutes. Stir in coconut milk, lime zest, lime juice, soy sauce and curry paste; bring to a boil. Reduce heat and simmer for 10 minutes or until sauce has thickened slightly. Season to taste with salt and pepper.

2. Ladle onto plates and garnish with cilantro.

PCOS Boost

Boost the nutrition of this recipe by adding 1 tbsp (15 mL) lecithin with the turkey. Sprinkle individual servings with dulse powder and ground flax seeds (flaxseed meal).

Turkey Apple Meatloaf

This yummy meatloaf boasts high fiber and healthy fat content, thanks to the oat bran and flax seeds. Add sunflower seeds, if desired.

Tips

Make extra turkey mixture and form into burger patties. After cooking, freeze in freezer bags for quick healthy lunches. Reheat burgers in the microwave on High for about 1 minute.

An extra meatloaf can be sliced to use in sandwiches or frozen for another day.

- Preheat oven to 350°F (180°C)
- 9- by 5-inch (23 by 12.5 cm) loaf pan, lightly greased

2	cloves garlic, minced	2
1	egg	1
1	tart apple, such as Mutsu or Granny Smith, finely chopped	1
1 lb	lean ground turkey	500 g
½ cup	chopped onion	125 mL
⅓ cup	oat bran	75 mL
⅓ cup	ground flax seeds (flaxseed meal)	75 mL
3 tbsp	prepared yellow mustard	45 mL
1 tbsp	ketchup	15 mL
1 tsp	salt	5 mL

1. In a large bowl, combine garlic, egg, apple, turkey, onion, oat bran, flax seeds, mustard, ketchup and salt. Pack into prepared loaf pan.

2. Bake in preheated oven for 45 to 60 minutes or until a meat thermometer inserted in the center registers an internal temperature of 175°F (80°C).

PCOS Boost

Boost the chromium content of this recipe by adding 2 tbsp (30 mL) lecithin and 2 tsp (10 mL) brewer's yeast.

Side Dishes

Oven-Roasted Asparagus

Makes 4 servings

Asparagus is not only delicious, it's also low on the glycemic index. It makes a great side with almost any meal — breakfast, lunch or dinner.

Tip

Roasting brings out the best in many vegetables, including asparagus. The oven-roasting method is much simpler and more flavorful than the traditional way of cooking asparagus in a steamer.

- Preheat oven to 425°F (220°C)
- Baking sheet, sprayed with vegetable cooking spray

1 lb	asparagus	500 g
1 tbsp	olive oil	15 mL
	Freshly ground black pepper	
1 tbsp	balsamic vinegar	15 mL

1. Snap off tough asparagus ends. If large, peel stalks. Arrange in single layer on prepared baking sheet. Drizzle with oil; season to taste with pepper.

2. Roast in oven, stirring occasionally, for 12 to 15 minutes or until almost tender.

3. Drizzle balsamic vinegar over asparagus and toss to coat. Roast for 3 to 5 minutes more or until tender-crisp. Serve immediately.

PCOS Boost

Boost the nutrition of this recipe by sprinkling individual servings with lecithin, nutritional yeast and crushed raw nuts.

Orange Broccoli

Makes 6 servings

Organic broccoli is available year-round. It makes an easy side for almost any meal.

Tips

Blanching enhances the colors of vegetables while maintaining their raw texture. To blanch vegetables, drop them into boiling water. Return to a boil and cook for 2 minutes. Drain and plunge into ice water.

If you don't have sunflower seeds on hand, substitute toasted nuts such as pine nuts, walnuts or almonds.

2 tbsp	freshly squeezed orange juice	30 mL
2 tsp	freshly squeezed lemon juice	10 mL
1 tbsp	vegetable oil	15 mL
1½ tsp	granulated sugar	7 mL
½ tsp	crushed dried basil	2 mL
¼ tsp	coarsely ground black pepper	1 mL
¼ tsp	Dijon mustard	1 mL
1	bunch broccoli florets, blanched, hot (see tip, at left)	1
2 tbsp	unsalted shelled sunflower seeds, toasted	30 mL

1. In a small bowl, whisk orange juice, lemon juice, oil, sugar, basil, pepper and mustard until blended.

2. Drizzle mixture over hot broccoli. Cover and let sauce heat until warm. Sprinkle with sunflower seeds.

PCOS Boost

Boost the nutrition of this recipe by substituting agave nectar or stevia powder for the sugar. Sprinkle individual servings with lecithin and nutritional yeast.

Ginger Carrots

Carrots are high on the glycemic index, but are so loaded with antioxidant nutrients, we'll forgive them.

Tip

Use the side of a spoon to scrape the skin off gingerroot before chopping or grating. Gingerroot keeps well in the freezer for up to 3 months and can be grated from frozen.

Variation

Substitute pure maple syrup, agave nectar or stevia powder for the brown sugar.

4 cups	chopped carrots	1 L
1/2 cup	vegetable or chicken broth	125 mL
2 tsp	minced gingerroot	10 mL
1 tsp	minced garlic	5 mL
1 tsp	packed brown sugar	5 mL
1/4 tsp	freshly squeezed lemon juice	1 mL

1. In a large saucepan, combine carrots, broth, ginger, garlic, brown sugar and lemon juice. Bring to a boil, then reduce heat, cover and simmer for about 20 minutes or until carrots are tender-crisp and liquid is absorbed.

PCOS Boost

Boost the nutrition of this recipe by sprinkling individual servings with lecithin, nutritional yeast and crushed raw nuts.

Golden Mushroom Sauté

Makes 8 servings

Mushrooms are very low on the glycemic index, and the flavorful sauce creates a fantastic dish.

Tip

To soften sun-dried tomatoes, cover with boiling water and let stand for 10 minutes. Drain well.

1 tsp	olive oil	5 mL
1	onion, chopped	1
2	cloves garlic, minced	2
1¼ lbs	chanterelle or portobello mushrooms, sliced	625 g
8 oz	small button mushrooms	250 g
3	sun-dried tomatoes, softened and chopped	3
¾ cup	chicken broth	175 mL
½ cup	dry white wine	125 mL
2 tbsp	freshly squeezed lemon juice	30 mL
1 tbsp	sweet Hungarian paprika	15 mL
½ tsp	caraway seeds	2 mL
	Salt and freshly ground black pepper	
2 tbsp	chopped fresh parsley	30 mL

1. In a large skillet, heat oil over medium heat; cook onion, stirring, for 2 minutes. Add garlic, chanterelle and button mushrooms and tomatoes; cook for 2 to 3 minutes.

2. Add chicken broth, wine, lemon juice, paprika and caraway seeds; bring to a boil. Simmer over low heat for about 15 minutes or until slightly thickened, stirring occasionally. Season to taste with salt and pepper. Sprinkle with parsley.

PCOS Boost

Boost the nutrition of this recipe by adding 1 tbsp (15 mL) prickly pear juice with the salt and pepper. Sprinkle individual servings with ground flax seeds (flaxseed meal), nutritional yeast and crushed raw nuts.

Fried Chinese Mushrooms

Don't let the fried aspect of this dish trouble you — when properly done, the mushrooms will be fairly low in fat. Be sure to use a heat-stable oil, such as walnut oil. Serve with cooked vegetables or a salad.

Tips

Five-spice powder is available in Asian markets or the specialty foods section of some supermarkets. Although dried shiitake mushrooms are available in most supermarkets, they are much more economical if purchased in Asian markets.

The secret to low-fat deep-frying is proper coating with cornstarch. If all of the mushroom is coated, very little fat will penetrate the food.

4	green onions	4
10	large dried shiitake mushrooms	10
½ cup	water	125 mL
4 tsp	cornstarch	20 mL
1 tsp	granulated sugar	5 mL
1 tsp	rice vinegar	5 mL
3½ tsp	tamari sauce or soy sauce	17 mL
¼ tsp	sesame oil	1 mL
Pinch	Chinese five-spice powder	Pinch
	Vegetable oil	
1	slice gingerroot	1
½	head iceberg lettuce, shredded	½

1. Cut green portion of onions lengthwise into slivers, without detaching from white part. Soak in bowl of water until slivers have curled. Soak mushrooms in medium bowl of water until soft, about 30 minutes.

2. Meanwhile, in a small saucepan, combine ½ cup (125 mL) water, 1 tsp (5 mL) of the cornstarch, sugar, vinegar, ½ tsp (2 mL) of the tamari sauce and sesame oil. Bring to a boil and cook until thickened; set aside.

3. Drain and rinse mushrooms; squeeze out excess water. Discard stems; slice caps into strips. Toss with 3 tsp (15 mL) of the tamari sauce; sprinkle with five-spice powder and toss to coat. Roll mushrooms in remaining cornstarch.

4. In a wok or frying pan, heat ¼ inch (5 mm) oil to 350°F (180°C). Fry gingerroot until lightly browned; discard. In small batches, fry mushroom strips until crisp, gently stirring with fork to prevent sticking. Drain on paper towels.

5. Place bed of lettuce on four individual plates. Warm sauce, then toss mushroom strips in sauce. Place strips on lettuce; drizzle with sauce. Garnish with curled green onion.

Italian Broiled Tomatoes

Makes 4 servings

This versatile, simple side dish complements a wide variety of meals, from fish and chicken to beans and casseroles.

Tip

Fresh tomatoes in season are a real treat. Store under-ripe tomatoes, unwashed, at room temperature away from sunlight until slightly soft. Room temperature tomatoes will have more flavor than cold ones.

- Preheat broiler
- Shallow baking pan

2	large tomatoes	2
Pinch	garlic powder	Pinch
1 tbsp	chopped fresh parsley	15 mL
1 tsp	dried basil	5 mL
½ tsp	dried oregano	2 mL
	Freshly ground black pepper	
2 tbsp	bread crumbs	30 mL

1. Cut tomatoes in half crosswise. Place cut side up on rack in shallow baking pan. Sprinkle lightly with garlic powder. Combine parsley, basil, oregano, pepper to taste and bread crumbs. Divide mixture over surface of tomato halves.

2. Place pan about 6 inches (15 cm) below broiler. Broil for 3 to 4 minutes, until tomatoes are heated through, or cook on barbecue along with meat being grilled.

PCOS Boost

Boost the nutrition of this recipe adding 1 tbsp (15 mL) lecithin and 1 tsp (5 mL) each dulse flakes and brewer's yeast to the parsley mixture. Substitute 1 tbsp (15 mL) each ground flax seeds (flaxseed meal) and nut flour for the bread crumbs. Sprinkle individual servings with nutritional yeast and sesame seeds or walnut pieces.

Braised Red Cabbage

	Makes 10 servings	

Braising brings out a **wonderful flavor from this dish. Cabbage is low on the glycemic index and is noted for its anticancer and hormone metabolizing effects.**

Tips

The apple and the red wine vinegar in this recipe add acid, which helps the cabbage keep its rich red color.

This dish reheats well and may be stored for 1 week in the refrigerator.

- Preheat oven to 325°F (160°C)
- 8-cup (2 L) baking dish

1	small red cabbage (about 1½ lb/750 g)	1
⅓ cup	red wine vinegar	75 mL
1 tbsp	granulated sugar	15 mL
1 tsp	salt	5 mL
1	slice bacon, chopped (or 1 tbsp/ 15 mL olive oil)	1
⅓ cup	chopped onion	75 mL
2	Granny Smith apples, peeled, cored and cut into eighths	2
1	whole clove	1
1	small onion	1
1	bay leaf	1
½ cup	boiling water	125 mL
2 tbsp	dry red wine (optional)	30 mL

1. Remove outer leaves of cabbage and discard. Cut cabbage into quarters; trim off excess white heart. Shred about ⅛ inch (3 mm) thick to make 6 cups (1.5 L). Place in bowl; toss with vinegar, sugar and salt.

2. In a large skillet, over medium heat, brown bacon; remove bacon, reserving drippings in pan. Set bacon aside. (If using oil, heat oil in skillet over medium heat.) Add chopped onion; cook, stirring, for 2 minutes. Add apples; cook for 5 minutes.

3. Push clove into onion; add to skillet along with cabbage mixture, bay leaf, boiling water and bacon. Mix well. Pour into 8-cup (2 L) baking dish. Cover and bake in preheated oven for 2 hours, stirring occasionally. (If it becomes dry, add more water.) Remove onion and bay leaf. Stir in wine, if desired.

PCOS Boost

Boost the nutrition of this recipe by substituting 1 tbsp (15 mL) agave nectar or 1 tsp (5 mL) stevia powder for the sugar. Sprinkle individual servings with raw nuts, ground flax seeds (flaxseed meal) and dulse flakes.

Stir-Fried Chinese Greens

Makes 6 servings		

Bok choy is a "super-green" because it is nutrient dense. Use a heat-stable oil, such as walnut oil, for sautéing.

1 tbsp	vegetable oil	15 mL
1	Spanish onion, cut lengthwise into thick slices	1
1	green bell pepper, julienned	1
1	head bok choy, cut into chunks (about 4 cups/1 L), white stalks and green leaves separated	1
1 cup	broccoli florets	250 mL
½ cup	water	125 mL
1 tbsp	hoisin sauce or your favorite stir-fry sauce	15 mL
2 tsp	reduced-sodium soy sauce	10 mL
½ tsp	sesame oil	2 mL
1 tbsp	sesame seeds	15 mL

1. Heat a wok or large skillet over medium heat. Add oil and swirl to coat. When oil is hot but not smoking, add onion and stir-fry for 3 minutes. Add green pepper and stir-fry for 2 minutes. Add white ends of the bok choy and the broccoli and stir-fry for 2 minutes. Stir in green bok choy leaves, water, hoisin sauce and soy sauce. Cover and cook for 3 minutes or until broccoli is tender-crisp.

2. Transfer to a serving dish, drizzle with sesame oil and sprinkle with sesame seeds.

PCOS Boost

Boost the nutrition of this recipe by sprinkling individual servings with nutritional yeast and dulse flakes.

Bitter Greens with Paprika

You can harvest your own dandelion greens for this dish; just make sure they haven't been sprayed with chemicals. Dandelion greens are extremely nutrient rich and help support healthy liver function. They are best in the spring months and become more bitter as the season continues.

1	bunch rapini or dandelion greens, bottom 2 inches (5 cm) of stalks trimmed	1
2 tbsp	olive oil	30 mL
1 tsp	sweet paprika	5 mL
1/4 tsp	ground turmeric	1 mL
1/4 tsp	salt	1 mL
1/4 tsp	freshly ground black pepper	1 mL
3	cloves garlic, thinly sliced	3
2 tbsp	freshly squeezed lemon juice	30 mL
1 tsp	drained capers	5 mL

1. Cut stalks of greens in half. Bring a pot of salted water to a boil and add the lower half of stalks. Let water return to boil and cook for 3 minutes. Add upper half of stalks (with the leaves); return to boil and cook for 3 minutes. Rinse under cold water; drain and set aside.

2. In a large frying pan, combine oil, paprika, turmeric, salt and pepper. Cook, stirring, over high heat for 1 minute. Add garlic; stir-fry for 30 seconds. Add drained greens; stir-fry for 2 minutes, folding from the bottom up to distribute garlic and spices evenly. Reduce heat to medium. Stir in lemon juice; cook, stirring, for 2 minutes. Stir in capers. Serve immediately.

PCOS Boost

Boost the nutrition of this recipe by adding 1 tbsp (15 mL) lecithin with the paprika. Sprinkle individual servings with raw nuts, nutritional yeast and ground flax seeds (flaxseed meal).

Sautéed Spinach with Pine Nuts

Spinach is very rich in fiber, antioxidants, vitamins and minerals, and combines well with almost any meal. Fresh organic spinach is usually available at well-stocked markets.

Tip

Stir-frying vegetables is a great way to preserve nutrients. When boiled, vegetables can lose up to 45% of vitamin C, compared with losing only 5% when stir-fried.

Variations

You can substitute Swiss chard, kale, rapini or mustard greens for the spinach.

If you don't have pine nuts, try pecans or walnuts.

2 tsp	olive oil	10 mL
¼ cup	pine nuts	60 mL
1	package (10 oz/300 g) fresh spinach, trimmed	1
1 tsp	minced garlic	5 mL
1 tsp	freshly squeezed lemon juice	5 mL
⅛ tsp	ground nutmeg	0.5 mL
	Freshly ground black pepper	

1. In a large nonstick skillet, heat 1 tsp (5 mL) of the oil over medium heat. Add pine nuts and cook, stirring constantly, for 2 to 3 minutes or until golden. Remove pine nuts from pan and set aside.

2. Add remaining oil to pan. Add spinach in several bunches (it will cook down quickly), stirring constantly. Add garlic and cook for 1 to 2 minutes. Stir in lemon juice and nutmeg. Season to taste with pepper. Add reserved pine nuts. Cook until heated through.

PCOS Boost

Boost the nutrition of this recipe by sprinkling individual servings with ground flax seeds (flaxseed meal) and nutritional yeast.

Spinach Fancy

Raisins, lemon and herbs are what make this spinach "fancy." Leftovers can be sautéed with eggs in the breakfast skillet or placed in a lunch box along with cooked fish or salad.

Tip

Use fresh herbs to replace any of the dried herbs in this recipe, but double or triple the amounts as the drying process intensifies the flavor of herbs.

1	package (10 oz/300 g) fresh spinach	1
3 tbsp	raisins	45 mL
Pinch	dried mint	Pinch
Pinch	ground fennel	Pinch
Pinch	dried oregano	Pinch
1 tbsp	butter or margarine	15 mL
2 tbsp	water	30 mL
1 tsp	freshly squeezed lemon juice	5 mL
1/2 tsp	salt	2 mL
Pinch	freshly ground black pepper	Pinch
	Lemon slices	

1. Wash spinach and dry thoroughly; remove stems and chop.

2. In a large skillet over medium heat, cook raisins, mint, fennel and oregano in butter. Add spinach and water; cover and steam for 2 to 3 minutes or until wilted. Drain liquid. Sprinkle with lemon juice, salt and pepper; toss well. Serve with lemon slices.

PCOS Boost

Boost the nutrition of this recipe by adding 1 tbsp (15 mL) lecithin and 1 tsp (5 mL) brewer's yeast with the raisins. Sprinkle individual servings with raw nuts, nutritional yeast and ground flax seeds (flaxseed meal).

Steamed Asian Vegetable Medley

The diverse vegetables in this dish offer a great deal of fiber, nutrients and antioxidant power. Steaming vegetables helps protect their valuable nutrients and flavor. A terrific addition to this dish would be edamame.

Tip

Choose organic vegetables whenever possible to reduce your exposure to harmful chemicals.

- **Steamer basket**

  Green vegetables: sugar snap peas, snow peas, finely chopped bok choy, chopped spinach

  Yellow/orange vegetables: baby corn, julienned yellow or orange bell peppers, yellow squash slices, carrot slices

  Red vegetables: julienned red bell peppers, cherry tomatoes, radishes

  White vegetables: bean sprouts, water chestnuts, turnip strips

  Sesame oil

  Soy sauce

  Toasted sesame seeds (optional)

1. In a medium saucepan, bring 1 cup (250 mL) water to a boil. Place steamer basket over boiling water and fill with vegetables. Drizzle with a small amount of sesame oil and soy sauce. Cover and steam until vegetables are tender-crisp.

2. Transfer to a serving dish and sprinkle with toasted sesame seeds, if desired.

Roasted Vegetables

Makes 8 servings

Roasting brings out a wonderful flavor from vegetables. You may omit the potatoes and the veggies that are high on the glycemic index. Use a heat-stable oil, such as walnut oil.

Tips

For the herbs, try any combination of thyme, oregano, basil, dill, parsley, chives and rosemary — whatever suits your taste! If you prefer, use 2 tsp (10 mL) dried herbs instead.

To save time, you can buy most veggies already cleaned and ready cut. The oil mixture can also be made a day in advance, covered and stored in the fridge.

These vegetables can also be grilled in a vegetable basket on a lightly greased barbecue preheated to medium. Cook, turning once, until tender, about 10 minutes.

- Preheat oven to 325°F (160°C)
- 13- by 9-inch (33 by 23 cm) roasting pan or shallow casserole dish, lightly greased

2	bell peppers (any color)	2
2	parsnips, peeled	2
2	carrots	2
2	potatoes (unpeeled)	2
1	onion	1
1	zucchini	1
1	bulb fennel	1
3	cloves garlic	3
2 tbsp	vegetable oil	30 mL
2 tbsp	pure maple syrup or liquid honey	30 mL
1 tbsp	Dijon mustard	15 mL
2 tbsp	chopped fresh herbs (see tip, at left)	30 mL
	Freshly ground black pepper	

1. Chop peppers, parsnips, carrots, potatoes, onion, zucchini and fennel into bite-size chunks. Spread vegetables and garlic in prepared pan.

2. In a medium bowl, combine oil, maple syrup, mustard and herbs. Pour over vegetables and toss to coat. Sprinkle with pepper to taste.

3. Roast in preheated oven, tossing once, for 30 to 40 minutes or until fork-tender and golden.

PCOS Boost

Boost the nutrition of this recipe by sprinkling individual servings with nutritional yeast and ground flax seeds (flaxseed meal).

Chickpea Curry

Makes 6 servings

This rich curry offers a serving of legumes in a flavorful vegetable base.

Tip

Use a heat-stable oil, such as walnut oil.

2 tbsp	vegetable oil	30 mL
¾ cup	diced onion	175 mL
1 tbsp	curry powder	15 mL
1 to 2 tbsp	all-purpose flour (or 1 tbsp/15 mL cornstarch)	15 to 30 mL
1 cup	water (approx.)	250 mL
⅔ cup	diced red bell pepper	150 mL
⅔ cup	diced yellow bell pepper	150 mL
1 cup	diced zucchini	250 mL
¾ cup	diced butternut squash	175 mL
1	can (19 oz/540 mL) chickpeas, drained and rinsed (about 2 cups/500 mL)	1
½ cup	vegetable broth	125 mL
½ cup	snow peas (optional)	125 mL
¼ cup	finely chopped fresh parsley (or 1 tbsp/15 mL dried)	60 mL

1. In a large skillet, heat oil over medium heat. Sauté onions until softened, about 5 minutes. Stir in curry powder. Sprinkle with 1 tbsp (15 mL) flour. Add water, stirring constantly to prevent lumping.

2. Add red and yellow peppers, zucchini and squash; bring to a boil. Cook, stirring often, for 10 minutes, adding more water if sauce is too thick. (If it's too thin, add the remaining flour, mixed with a little water.)

3. Add chickpeas and broth; reduce heat and simmer for 10 minutes, until chickpeas are heated through. Add snow peas (if using) and parsley just before serving.

PCOS Boost

Boost the nutrition of this recipe by sprinkling individual servings with nutritional yeast, ground flax seeds (flaxseed meal) and raw nuts.

Easy Black Beans

Black beans help stabilize blood sugar levels and, like all legumes, provide protein and fiber, which can improve cholesterol levels and hormone regulation.

Tip

If your family doesn't like heat, leave out the chipotle pepper.

1 tsp	vegetable oil	5 mL
1	small onion, chopped	1
1	can (19 oz/540 mL) black beans, drained and rinsed (about 2 cups/500 mL)	1
1½ cups	water	375 mL
½ cup	tomato paste	125 mL
1	chipotle pepper in adobo sauce	1
1	bay leaf	1
1 tsp	ground cumin	5 mL
2 tbsp	chopped fresh cilantro (optional)	30 mL

1. In a large skillet, heat oil over medium heat. Sauté onion until softened, about 5 minutes. Stir in beans, water, tomato paste, chipotle pepper, bay leaf and cumin; bring to a boil. Reduce heat and simmer for 15 minutes or until slightly thickened. Discard the chipotle and bay leaf. (If you leave the chipotle in, the dish will be too spicy)!

2. Ladle into bowls and garnish with cilantro, if desired.

PCOS Boost

Boost the chromium content of this recipe by adding 1 tsp (5 mL) lecithin and ¼ tsp (1 mL) brewer's yeast.

Desserts

Broiled Nectarines

Quick to prepare and extremely satisfying, this fruit dessert makes a nice winter or cold weather choice.

Variations

Substitute pears for the nectarines

Substitute 2 grapefruit, cut in half, for the nectarines and omit the yogurt.

Substitute cottage cheese for the yogurt.

- 9-inch (23 cm) square casserole dish
- 4 small custard cups or dessert cups

2	nectarines	2
2 tbsp	granulated date sugar	30 mL
2 tbsp	pure maple syrup	30 mL
2 tbsp	orange-flavored liqueur (such as Grand Marnier)	30 mL
1 tbsp	canola oil	15 mL
1 tsp	freshly grated nutmeg	5 mL
1 cup	low-fat vanilla-flavored yogurt, divided	250 mL
	Raspberries and/or blueberries (optional)	

1. Cut nectarines in half lengthwise and twist halves to separate; remove pits. Place nectarines rounded side down in casserole dish.

2. In a small bowl, combine date sugar, maple syrup, liqueur, oil and nutmeg. Spoon on top of nectarines. Let stand at room temperature for 20 minutes.

3. Meanwhile, preheat broiler, with rack set 4 inches (10 cm) from heat.

4. Broil nectarines for 6 to 7 minutes or until topping is bubbling and caramelized.

5. Spoon nectarines and any liquid into ramekins and spoon yogurt on top. Garnish with berries (if using).

Desserts and PCOS

While desserts aren't ideal for your nutritional and metabolic goals, there will always be special occasions when you may want one. The 10 recipes in this chapter are healthier than most because they are based on sweet fruits rather than sugar, and offer some nutritional value rather than empty calories. Nevertheless, desserts are best reserved for special occasions and consumed in small quantities.

Spiced Carrot Cake with Currants

Makes 16 servings

In this healthy version of a dessert classic, the nuts and rolled oats replace some of the flour, to keep the glycemic index down. And the carrots offer beta carotene and other valuable nutrients.

Tip

Store the cooled cake at room temperature in a cake keeper, or loosely wrapped in foil or plastic wrap, for up to 3 days. Alternatively, wrap it in plastic wrap, then foil, completely enclosing cake, and freeze for up to 6 months. Let thaw at room temperature for 4 to 6 hours before serving.

- Preheat oven to 325°F (160°C)
- Food processor
- 9-inch (23 cm) square metal baking pan, sprayed with nonstick baking spray with flour

1 cup	quick-cooking rolled oats	250 mL
1 cup	chopped walnuts or pecans	250 mL
1 cup	whole wheat pastry flour	250 mL
2 tsp	baking powder	10 mL
1 tsp	baking soda	5 mL
1 tsp	ground cinnamon	5 mL
½ tsp	ground ginger	2 mL
½ tsp	fine sea salt	2 mL
2 cups	shredded carrots	500 mL
⅔ cup	dried currants	150 mL
½ cup	unsweetened flaked coconut	125 mL
1 cup	pure maple syrup, brown rice syrup or liquid honey	250 mL
2 tsp	vanilla extract	10 mL

1. In food processor, combine oats and walnuts; pulse until coarsely ground.

2. In a large bowl, whisk together oat mixture, flour, baking powder, baking soda, cinnamon, ginger and salt.

3. In a medium bowl, combine carrots, currants, coconut, maple syrup and vanilla.

4. Add the carrot mixture to the flour mixture and stir with a wooden spoon until blended.

5. Spread batter evenly in prepared pan.

6. Bake in preheated oven for 50 to 60 minutes or until a toothpick inserted in the center comes out with a few moist crumbs attached. Let cool completely in pan on a wire rack.

Five-Minute Cheesecake Cups with Raspberries

Each serving of this super-simple dessert contains only 1½ tsp (7 mL) of sweetener. Berries are high in antioxidants, and the cottage cheese and pistachios make this dessert high in protein.

- Food processor
- Two 6-oz (175 mL) ramekins or dessert glasses

1 cup	nonfat cottage cheese	250 mL
1 tbsp	agave nectar or liquid honey	15 mL
½ tsp	vanilla extract	2 mL
⅔ cup	raspberries	150 mL
2 tbsp	finely chopped lightly salted roasted pistachios	30 mL

1. In food processor, combine cottage cheese, agave nectar and vanilla; purée until smooth.

2. Divide mixture between ramekins. Top with raspberries and pistachios.

Minted Fruit Salad

This dessert is especially nice in the summer, when you can take advantage of locally grown fresh fruit and mint. Berries are high in powerful antioxidants that have been shown to reduce inflammatory processes in the blood and blood vessels.

1½ cups	quartered hulled strawberries	375 mL
1½ cups	blackberries	375 mL
1 cup	fresh pineapple chunks	250 mL
1 cup	diced kiwifruit	250 mL
1 cup	loosely packed mint leaves, chopped	250 mL
1 tbsp	freshly squeezed lemon juice	15 mL
1 tbsp	agave nectar or liquid honey	15 mL

1. In a large bowl, gently toss strawberries, blackberries, pineapple, kiwi, mint, lemon juice and agave nectar. Serve within 1 to 2 hours.

Honey-Roasted Plums with Ricotta

Fruit and cheese always taste great together. With only 1½ tsp (7 mL) of honey per serving, this delicious dessert is a fairly innocent sweet.

- Preheat oven to 400°F (200°C)
- Large rimmed baking sheet, lined with parchment paper

8	large red or purple plums, each cut into 8 wedges	8
2 tbsp	liquid honey, divided	30 mL
1⅓ cups	nonfat ricotta cheese	325 mL
2 tbsp	chopped toasted walnuts	30 mL

1. In a medium bowl, gently toss plums and half the honey. Arrange in a single layer on prepared baking sheet.

2. Roast in preheated oven for 15 to 20 minutes or until browned at the edges. Let cool completely on pan.

3. In a small bowl, combine cheese and the remaining honey.

4. Divide cheese mixture among four dessert dishes. Top with roasted plums and walnuts.

Goat Cheese and Pistachio–Stuffed Dates

Makes 8 servings

This simple dessert works well at parties as finger food, placed on a tray with fresh fruit slices.

8 tsp	soft goat cheese	40 mL
1 tbsp	finely chopped lightly salted roasted pistachios	15 mL
8	large Medjool dates, pitted	8

1. In a small bowl, combine cheese and pistachios.

2. Stuff each date with a heaping teaspoon (5 mL) of the cheese mixture.

Fresh Figs and Melon with Blue Cheese

Makes 6 servings		

This unusual dessert is easy to prepare and contains only a small amount of agave nectar, for a touch of sweetness.

Tips

A cantaloupe that is very hard and does not yield much to firm pressure may be under-ripe. A cantaloupe that yields greatly to firm pressure or has indentations may be over-ripe. Try smelling the stem scar: a ripe cantaloupe will smell sweeter and more aromatic then an under-ripe one.

Crush pecans by placing them in a small sealable plastic bag and rolling them with a rolling pin.

Any leftover yogurt dressing can be refrigerated for 1 day in an airtight container.

	Grated zest and juice of 1 lime	
1 cup	nonfat or low-fat vanilla-flavored yogurt	250 mL
2 tbsp	agave nectar	30 mL
12	figs, stems removed, cut in half lengthwise	12
1/2	small cantaloupe, scooped into balls or cubed	1/2
	Seeds of 1/2 pomegranate	
1 cup	crumbled blue cheese	250 mL
1/4 cup	crushed pecans	60 mL
1/4 cup	fresh mint leaves, finely chopped (optional)	60 mL

1. In a small bowl, combine lime zest, lime juice, yogurt and agave nectar. Cover and refrigerate until serving, for up to 1 day.

2. Arrange 4 fig halves on each of six individual plates or in small, shallow bowls. Divide cantaloupe and pomegranate seeds equally among plates. Drizzle yogurt dressing on top and sprinkle with blue cheese, pecans and mint (if using).

Cocoa Truffles

Makes 2 dozen truffles

Truffles with no sugar! This simple recipe uses dates as a sweetener and easily satisfies a chocolate craving.

Tip

Store the truffles in an airtight container in the refrigerator for up to 1 week.

- Food processor

2 cups	pecan halves	500 mL
	Cold water	
2 cups	packed chopped pitted dates	500 mL
2/3 cup	unsweetened cocoa powder (preferably natural cocoa)	150 mL
1/4 tsp	fine sea salt	1 mL
1 tbsp	vanilla extract	15 mL

1. Place pecans in a medium bowl and add enough cold water to cover. Let soak for 4 to 6 hours to soften. Drain well.

2. In food processor, pulse softened pecans until chopped. Add dates, cocoa powder, salt and vanilla; process until almost smooth, stopping once or twice to scrape sides of bowl.

3. Transfer pecan mixture to a medium bowl. Cover and refrigerate for at least 2 hours or until firm enough to roll.

4. Roll pecan mixture into 1-inch (2.5 cm) balls.

Vanilla Cashew Ice Cream

Makes 4 servings

Ice cream lovers rejoice. This unusual dairy-free "ice cream" uses cashews to create the creamy texture and provide healthy fats.

- Blender
- Ice cream maker

1 cup	raw cashews	250 mL
1/8 tsp	fine sea salt	0.5 mL
2 cups	ice water	500 mL
1/4 cup	agave nectar or liquid honey	60 mL
1 tbsp	vanilla extract	15 mL

1. In blender, combine cashews, salt, ice water, agave nectar and vanilla; purée on high speed for 2 minutes.

2. Pour into ice cream maker and freeze according to manufacturer's instructions.

3. Spoon into an airtight container, cover and freeze for 4 hours, until firm, or for up to 3 days.

Ricotta Pudding with Strawberry Coulis

Makes 6 servings

Eggs and ricotta provide protein, and the fresh strawberries make this dessert a rather innocent sweet.

Tip

Choose strawberries that look plump and glossy; dull ones are usually past their prime. Store strawberries in the refrigerator in a container with air holes for up to 3 days. Bring them to room temperature for the best flavor.

- Preheat oven to 375°F (190°C)
- Blender or food processor
- 9-inch (23 cm) glass pie plate, sprayed with nonstick cooking spray (preferably olive oil)

3	large eggs	3
2 cups	nonfat ricotta cheese	500 mL
4 tbsp	liquid honey, divided	60 mL
2 tsp	vanilla extract	10 mL
1/8 tsp	fine sea salt	0.5 mL
2 cups	quartered hulled strawberries	500 mL
1 tbsp	water	15 mL
2 tsp	balsamic vinegar	10 mL

1. In blender, combine eggs, ricotta, 3 tbsp (45 mL) of the honey, vanilla and salt; purée for 1 to 2 minutes or until very smooth. Pour into prepared pie plate.

2. Bake in preheated oven for 22 to 26 minutes or until golden and just set at the center. Let cool on a wire rack.

3. Meanwhile, in clean blender, combine strawberries, the remaining honey, water and vinegar; purée until smooth. Cover and refrigerate for at least 30 minutes, until chilled, or for up to 1 day.

4. Cut pudding into wedges and serve with strawberry coulis.

Medicinal Beverages

Prickly Pear Power Punch

This is featured frequently in the weekly meal plans (pages 146–153) as an example of how to get the nutrients recommended for treating PCOS. It's easy and delicious, and should be consumed frequently to help regain hormonal and metabolic balance.

Variation

Use cold brewed hibiscus tea (see tip, page 249) or a blend of hibiscus tea and Stevia Tea (page 254) in place of water.

1 tsp	inositol powder	5 mL
1 tbsp	prickly pear juice	15 mL
1	drop vitamin D3 liquid (see tip, page 265)	1
2 cups	cold spring water or sparkling mineral water	500 mL
	Citrus slice (optional)	

1. In a tall glass, combine inositol powder, prickly pear juice and vitamin D; stir into a paste. Add water and stir to blend well. Drink immediately.

Fruit Juice and PCOS

Many people take in a great deal of carbohydrates in the form of beverages — soda pop, super-sweetened lattes, "energy drinks" and poor-quality fruit punches loaded with corn syrup and other simple sugars. Even some pure, good-quality fruit juices have a high glycemic index when stripped of their fiber and consumed in large quantities. Therefore, fruit juices are discouraged for those with insulin resistance and PCOS. Especially to be avoided are juices to which sweeteners and corn syrup are added. One way to enjoy fruit juices and stay on a healthy diet is to make sure all the fiber is blended into the drink. Another is to prepare fresh fruit-flavored water, such as the recipes on pages 247–248.

Agua de Manzana (Apple Water)

My time in Peru has given me an appreciation for the subtle and refreshing flavors of fruit waters. The preparation couldn't be simpler. Make a pitcher every morning, refrigerate and watch it disappear.

Tips

For the best flavor, choose tart apples, such as Jonathan or Granny Smith.

In Peru, people leave the cores, seeds and apple pieces in the water and let them settle on the bottom of the pitcher, decanting just the water as they pour. If this troubles you, strain out the solids after the flavor has infused for 2 or 3 hours, then refrigerate the strained water.

Choose organic apples whenever possible. Pesticides, herbicides and other chemicals used on non-organic produce burden the liver and can add to hormonal and metabolic imbalances.

2	apples	2
8 cups	spring water	2 L
	Prickly pear juice	

1. Cut apples into small chunks and place in a pitcher (you can include the core, seeds and/or skin, if desired). Add spring water. Cover and refrigerate for about 2 hours, until chilled and flavor is infused, or for up to 2 days.

2. To serve, pour water into a glass and add 1 to 3 tsp (5 to 15 mL) prickly pear juice, to taste.

Minty Lemon Water

This mint- and citrus-infused water is very refreshing on a hot day.

2	lemons	2
1 cup	packed fresh mint leaves, chopped	250 mL
8 cups	spring water or sparkling mineral water	2 L
	Prickly pear juice (optional)	

1. Grate the zest of the lemons into a pitcher. Cut lemons in half crosswise and squeeze the juice into the pitcher, straining through a fine-mesh sieve, if desired, to catch seeds and pulp. Discard seeds and add any pulp to the pitcher. Add mint and spring water. Cover and refrigerate for about 2 hours, until chilled and flavor is infused, or for up to 1 day.

2. To serve, pour water into a glass and add 1 to 3 tsp (5 to 15 mL) prickly pear juice, to taste (if using).

Tips

You can leave the lemon pieces and mint in the water and let them settle on the bottom of the pitcher, decanting just the water as you pour. If this troubles you, strain out the solids after the flavor has infused for 2 or 3 hours, then refrigerate the strained water.

Use organic lemons for this drink if you can find them. If the lemons have been sprayed, using the zest will put unwanted chemicals in your beverage.

Variation

Replace the lemons with oranges or 1 cup (250 mL) chopped watermelon, cantaloupe or honeydew melon or 1 star fruit, cut into thin slices.

Prickly Pear Spritzer

Prickly pear is a wonderful fruit for improving insulin resistance and reducing blood sugars and fats. Use it on a daily basis wherever you can.

1 to 2	limes	1 to 2
5 to 6	frozen cranberries (optional)	5 to 6
1 cup	Stevia Tea (page 254), chilled	250 mL
1 cup	sparkling mineral water	250 mL
¼ cup	prickly pear juice	60 mL

1. Using a zester, remove the zest of 1 lime in long strips, avoiding the white pith. Squeeze juice from lime(s) to obtain ¼ cup (60 mL).

2. In a large glass, combine lime zest and cranberries (if using). Stir in lime juice, stevia tea, mineral water and prickly pear juice. Serve immediately.

Blueberry Spritzer

Both prickly pear and blueberries help protect the blood vessels from the damaging effects of high blood glucose and cholesterol.

Tip

To make hibiscus tea, in a teapot combine 1 tbsp (15 mL) dried hibiscus flowers and 1 cup (250 mL) boiling water. Cover and let steep for 10 to 15 minutes. Strain through a tea strainer or fine-mesh sieve. Refrigerate for about 2 hours, until chilled, or for up to 2 days.

- **Blender**

1 tbsp	inositol powder	15 mL
2 cups	unsweetened blueberry juice, chilled	500 mL
1 cup	hibiscus tea, chilled (see tip, at left)	250 mL
¼ cup	prickly pear juice	60 mL
1 cup	sparkling mineral water, chilled	250 mL

1. In blender, combine inositol powder, blueberry juice, hibiscus tea and prickly pear juice; purée until smooth. Using a spoon, stir in mineral water.

2. Pour into glasses and serve cold.

Sparkling Aloe Hibiscus Spritzer

Makes 2 to 3 servings		

This cooling, soothing beverage is great on a hot day.

Tip

If using fresh aloe, be sure the plant has not been sprayed with insecticides or fungicides. Commercially prepared, food-grade aloe gel is available in health food stores.

- Blender

2 tbsp	dried hibiscus flowers (see tip, page 255)	30 mL
1 tbsp	dried stevia leaves	15 mL
3 cups	boiling spring water	750 mL
1 tbsp	peeled fresh aloe pulp or commercial aloe gel	15 mL
	Grated zest and juice of 1 orange	
3 cups	sparkling mineral water	750 mL

1. In a teapot or saucepan, combine hibiscus flowers and stevia leaves. Pour in boiling water, cover and let steep for 20 minutes. Strain through a tea strainer or fine-mesh sieve into a bowl or container. Refrigerate for about 4 hours or until chilled.

2. In blender, combine hibiscus tea, aloe, orange zest and orange juice; purée until smooth. Pour into a pitcher and stir in mineral water. Serve immediately.

Fruit Vinegar Spritzers

Makes 1 serving		

You'll be amazed by how delicious and un-vinegar-like this drink is.

Tip

Look for fruit vinegars, such as raspberry, blueberry or grapefruit, in gourmet shops and well-stocked supermarkets.

1 tbsp	fruit vinegar	15 mL
	Ice cubes	
3 to 4	frozen cranberries or blueberries	3 to 4
1 tbsp	prickly pear juice (optional)	15 mL
2 cups	sparkling mineral water	500 mL
	Lemon slice	

1. Place fruit vinegar in a tall glass. Add several ice cubes, frozen berries and prickly pear juice (if using). Fill the glass with mineral water. Garnish with a lemon slice and serve immediately.

Pomegranate Apricot Fizz

Pomegranates are high in antioxidants and anti-inflammatory flavonoids, and inositol powder and prickly pear help improve insulin resistance.

1	lemon	1
1 tbsp	inositol powder	15 mL
1 cup	unsweetened apricot nectar	250 mL
2 cups	sparkling mineral water	500 mL
2 cups	unsweetened pomegranate juice	500 mL
1/4 cup	prickly pear juice	60 mL

1. Using a zester, remove zest from lemon in long strips, avoiding the white pith. Squeeze juice from lemon to obtain 1/4 cup (60 mL).

2. Place inositol powder in a pitcher. Pour in apricot nectar, vigorously stirring as you pour. Stir in lemon juice, mineral water, pomegranate juice and prickly pear juice.

3. Pour into glasses and garnish with lemon zest.

Jalapeño Punch

Makes 2 to 3 servings

This is an unusual punch for spice lovers. It is sweet, sour and spicy all at once.

Tip

The heat level in jalapeño peppers varies, so you may want to add more or less than 1 tbsp (15 mL). If the pepper you have seems very hot, start with a little less and taste the juice after it has steeped for a couple of hours. You can always add more to boost the heat. If the pepper you have seems mild, add a little more than 1 tbsp (15 mL).

1 1/2 tbsp	dried hibiscus flowers (see tip, page 255)	22 mL
3 cups	boiling water	750 mL
1 tsp	inositol powder	5 mL
2 tbsp	agave nectar	30 mL
1 tbsp	thin strips seeded jalapeño pepper (see tip, at left)	15 mL
1 cup	fresh mint leaves, finely snipped	250 mL
2 cups	sparkling mineral water, chilled	500 mL
1 cup	ice cubes	250 mL

1. Place hibiscus flowers in a teapot or saucepan. Pour in boiling water, cover and let steep for 10 minutes. Strain through a tea strainer or fine-mesh sieve into a container. Stir in inositol powder and agave nectar until dissolved.

2. Place jalapeño and mint in a pitcher. Pour in warm tea and stir. Cover and refrigerate for 8 hours, until chilled, or overnight.

3. Just before serving, stir in mineral water. Place ice cubes in glasses and pour punch over top.

Spicy Tomato Juice

Makes 4 to
5 servings

Good for what ails you,
this is a nourishing
drink, and the
addition of garlic,
ginger, onions and
lecithin boosts the
medicinal value. The
seaweed — very rich
in minerals, including
iodine — may support
thyroid function.

Tip

Store any leftover juice
in the blender jug in the
refrigerator. Blend again
before serving and use
within the day.

● **Blender**

2	cloves garlic	2
¼ cup	coarsely chopped onion	60 mL
2 tsp	chopped fresh gingerroot	10 mL
1 tsp	minced seeded habanero pepper	5 mL
2 tsp	lecithin granules or liquid	10 mL
½ to 1 tsp	dulse or other seaweed granules or powder	2 to 5 mL
½ tsp	celery salt	2 mL
½ tsp	brewer's yeast	2 mL
1 tbsp	grated lemon zest	15 mL
½ cup	freshly squeezed lemon juice	125 mL
1 tbsp	flaxseed oil	15 mL
1 tsp	prepared horseradish	5 mL
4 cups	unsalted tomato juice, chilled	1 L
	Thin celery stalks	

1. In blender, combine garlic, onion, ginger, habanero
   pepper, lecithin, dulse to taste, celery salt, brewer's
   yeast, lemon zest, lemon juice, flaxseed oil and
   horseradish; purée until smooth. Add tomato juice
   and blend until incorporated.

2. Pour into tall glasses and garnish with celery.

Almond Milk

This delicious milk substitute is easy to make and has no saturated fat and no cholesterol.

Tips

This recipe will not work with toasted or roasted almonds. Be sure to use raw almonds.

If desired, add agave nectar to taste to each serving of almond milk.

Variation

For a sweeter version, replace the boiling water with hot stevia tea. To prepare 6 cups (1.5 L) stevia tea, combine 4 tsp (20 mL) dried stevia leaves with 6 cups (1.5 L) boiling water.

- Blender
- Jelly bag or sieve lined with cheesecloth (optional)

3 cups	raw almonds	750 mL
6 cups	boiling spring water	1.5 L
6 cups	spring water	1.5 L

1. Place almonds in blender and pour in boiling water. Cover and let stand at least overnight or for 24 hours, if possible. The almonds will swell overnight and soak up a good deal of the water.

2. Add fresh spring water and purée as finely as possible (if your blender won't hold this volume, remove half or two-thirds of the soaked almonds, then purée with the water in two or three batches).

3. If you like, you may leave the fine nut particulate in the milk if you are going to use it to make a smoothie or pour it over oatmeal or fresh fruit. To strain, pour almond purée into a jelly bag or cheesecloth-lined sieve and strain the liquid to remove all particulate (use the particulate elsewhere, if desired, such as in muffin recipes, or freeze for later use). Store almond milk in an airtight container in the refrigerator for up to 2 days.

Warm Almond Nutmeg Milk

Makes 2 servings

This warm, nicely spiced beverage works well as a breakfast or as dessert on a chilly evening.

Variation

As an occasional indulgence, add a shot of espresso to the mug before adding the warm milk.

3 tbsp	maca powder	45 mL
2 tsp	arrowroot powder	10 mL
1 tsp	inositol powder	5 mL
1/2 tsp	brewer's yeast	2 mL
1 tbsp	agave nectar	15 mL
1/2 tsp	walnut oil	2 mL
3 cups	Almond Milk (page 253)	750 mL
1/2 tsp	freshly grated nutmeg (or 1/4 tsp/1 mL ground)	2 mL

1. In a saucepan, combine maca powder and arrowroot powder. Stir in inositol powder, brewer's yeast, agave nectar and walnut oil. Using a fork, stir in 1 to 2 tbsp (15 to 30 mL) of the almond milk to thoroughly moisten the powder and avoid lumps. Gradually stir in the remaining almond milk.

2. Place saucepan over low heat and bring milk mixture to a very gentle simmer, stirring often. Remove from heat and stir for 3 to 4 minutes or until arrowroot begins to thicken the milk. Ladle into mugs and stir half the nutmeg into each serving.

Stevia Tea

Makes 1 cup (250 mL)

Stevia tea is used as a sweetener in many of these beverage recipes. You can use it hot or cold.

1 tsp	dried stevia leaves	5 mL
1 cup	boiling water	250 mL

1. In a teapot or measuring cup, combine stevia leaves and boiling water. Cover and let steep for 10 minutes. Strain through a tea strainer or fine-mesh sieve. Use hot or refrigerate until chilled.

Summer Tea

**This tea provides
a great deal of
chromium and is
cooling and refreshing.
Hibiscus is the highest
known source of
chromium, and all
of these herbs help
balance blood sugar.**

Tip

Dried hibiscus flowers are
available in herb shops
and health food stores.
If you can't find them, use
2 commercial tea bags
that have hibiscus as a
main ingredient.

1 cup	dried stevia leaves	250 mL
1 cup	dried hibiscus flowers (see tip, at left)	250 mL
1 cup	dried chopped lemongrass	250 mL
1 cup	dried nettle leaves	250 mL

To Serve

Boiling water

1. In a jar or sealable plastic bag, combine stevia leaves, hibiscus flowers, lemongrass and nettle leaves. Seal and store in a cool, dry place for up to 1 year.

2. *To serve:* For each serving, place 1 tbsp (15 mL) herb mixture in a teapot and pour in 1 cup (250 mL) boiling water. Cover and let steep for 10 minutes. Strain through a tea strainer or fine-mesh sieve into a mug and serve hot. Alternatively, strain into a container, refrigerate until chilled and serve cold or over ice.

Herbal Teas

Herbal teas are a great way to consume herbs for medicinal effects. Although they may be weaker than some highly concentrated herbal pills, they are relatively inexpensive, provide minerals and some nutrients, and are an opportunity for relaxation and self-nurturing. Brew up a pot, light a candle and curl up with a good book. Drinking these teas day after day can provide a significant medicinal effect. Herbal teas have little to no calories and can help increase your fluid intake.

Winter Tea

These blood sugar–balancing herbs make a warming welcome drink on a chilly day.

Tips

Licorice root may be available in several forms in herb shops: long thin slices of whole root, roots chopped into pea-sized or smaller chunks, or very finely shredded roots (sometimes called "tea cut"). For best results, choose shredded roots. If they're not available, coarsely chopped will do.

Astragalus roots may be available in a couple of forms in herb shops: long thin slices of whole root that look like tongue depressors, or very finely shredded roots (sometimes called "tea cut"). For making herbal teas, choose shredded astragalus roots.

1 cup	shredded dried licorice root	250 mL
1 cup	small pieces cinnamon bark	250 mL
1 cup	fenugreek seeds	250 mL
1 cup	shredded dried astragalus root	250 mL

To Serve

Boiling water

1. In a jar or sealable plastic bag, combine licorice root, cinnamon bark, fenugreek seeds and astragalus root. Seal and store in a cool, dry place for up to 1 year.

2. *To serve:* For each serving, place 1 tsp (5 mL) herb mixture in a teapot and pour in 1 cup (250 mL) boiling water. Cover and let steep for 10 minutes. Strain through a tea strainer or fine-mesh sieve into a mug and serve hot.

Hibiscus Herb Tea

**Makes about
4 cups (1 L)
herb mixture**

This tea helps improve insulin resistance, is high in chromium and offers many nutrients.

Tip

It is important to drink this tea the day it is made.

2 cups	dried alfalfa leaves	500 mL
1 cup	dried stevia leaves	250 mL
1 cup	dried hibiscus flowers (see tip, page 255)	250 mL

To Serve

Boiling water

1. In a jar or sealable plastic bag, combine alfalfa leaves, stevia leaves and hibiscus flowers. Seal and store in a cool, dry place for up to 1 year.

2. *To serve:* For each serving, place 1 tbsp (15 mL) herb mixture in a teapot and pour in 1 cup (250 mL) boiling water. Cover and let steep for 10 to 15 minutes, until desired strength. Strain through a tea strainer or fine-mesh sieve into a mug and serve hot.

Medicinal Mint Tea

**Makes about
3 cups (750 mL)
herb mixture**

This tea helps improve insulin resistance, thanks to its high chromium content, offers a good deal of nutrients and is hormone balancing.

Tip

It is important to drink this tea the day it is made.

1 cup	dried peppermint leaves	250 mL
1 cup	dried alfalfa leaves	250 mL
1/2 cup	dried stevia leaves	125 mL
1/2 cup	dried hibiscus flowers (see tip, page 255)	125 mL

To Serve

Boiling water

1. In a jar or sealable plastic bag, combine peppermint leaves, alfalfa leaves, stevia leaves and hibiscus flowers. Seal and store in a cool, dry place for up to 1 year.

2. *To serve:* For each serving, place 1 tbsp (15 mL) herb mixture in a teapot and pour in 1 cup (250 mL) boiling water. Cover and let steep for 10 to 15 minutes, until desired strength. Strain through a tea strainer or fine-mesh sieve into a mug and serve hot.

Astragalus Tea

This tea is warming
in the winter and
supports healthy blood
sugar, fat metabolism
and immune function.

Tip

It is important to drink this
tea the day it is made.

2 cups	shredded dried astragalus root	500 mL
1 cup	shredded dried licorice root	250 mL
½ cup	shredded dried gingerroot	125 mL
¼ cup	fenugreek seeds	60 mL

To Serve

Boiling water

1. In a jar or sealable plastic bag, combine astragalus root, licorice root, ginger and fenugreek seeds. Seal and store in a cool, dry place for up to 1 year.

2. *To serve:* For each serving, place 1 tsp (5 mL) herb mixture in a teapot and pour in 1 cup (250 mL) boiling water. Cover and let steep for 10 to 15 minutes, until desired strength. Strain through a tea strainer or fine-mesh sieve into a mug and serve hot.

Cinnamon Tea

Cinnamon is aromatic
and delicious, and
supports healthy
circulation and blood
sugar regulation to
boot. Cinnamon tea
is especially nice in
the morning or on
chilly days, as it has a
warming effect.

Tip

It is important to drink this
tea the day it is made.

1 cup	shredded dried astragalus root	250 mL
1 cup	small chunks cinnamon bark	250 mL
1 cup	shredded or small chunks Oregon grape root	250 mL
1 cup	shredded dried licorice root	250 mL

To Serve

Boiling water

1. In a jar or sealable plastic bag, combine astragalus root, cinnamon, grape root and licorice root. Seal and store in a cool, dry place for up to 1 year.

2. *To serve:* For each serving, place 1 tsp (5 mL) herb mixture in a teapot and pour in 1 cup (250 mL) boiling water. Cover and let steep for 10 to 15 minutes, until desired strength. Strain through a tea strainer or fine-mesh sieve into a mug and serve hot.

Elderberry Tea

**This tea supports
healthy metabolism
of blood sugar and
fats and has immune-
boosting effects. Brew
it up if you feel like
you might be coming
down with a cold.**

Tips

It is important to drink this tea the day it is made.

Make a large batch of tea to consume over the day using 6 to 8 tsp (30 to 40 mL) of the herb blend and 6 to 8 cups (1.5 to 2 L) water. Place the strained tea in a Thermos to keep it warm, reheat on the stovetop or in the microwave as desired, or enjoy cold or at room temperature.

½ cup	dried elderberries	125 mL
½ cup	shredded dried astragalus root	125 mL
½ cup	shredded dried licorice root	125 mL
½ cup	small chunks cinnamon bark	125 mL
½ cup	shredded dried gingerroot	125 mL

To Serve

Boiling water

1. In a jar or sealable plastic bag, combine elderberries, astragalus root, licorice root, cinnamon and ginger. Seal and store in a cool, dry place for up to 1 year.

2. *To serve:* For each serving, place 1 tsp (5 mL) herb mixture in a teapot and pour in 1 cup (250 mL) boiling water. Cover and let steep for 10 to 15 minutes, until desired strength. Strain through a tea strainer or fine-mesh sieve into a mug and serve hot.

Flor de Jamaica Tea

Hibiscus is called *flor de Jamaica* in some parts of Latin America. This tea, with its beautiful red color, is a traditional holiday beverage.

⅓ cup	dried hibiscus flowers (see tip, page 255)	75 mL
2 tbsp	dried stevia leaves	30 mL
¼ cup	sliced fresh gingerroot	60 mL
6 cups	boiling water	1.5 L
1	orange, cut into round slices	1

1. In a saucepan or teapot, combine hibiscus flowers, stevia and ginger. Pour in boiling water, cover and let steep for 20 minutes. Strain through a fine-mesh sieve into a pitcher or container and refrigerate for at least 4 hours, until chilled, or for up to 1 day.

2. Pour chilled tea into glasses and garnish with an orange slice on the rim.

Warm Mulled Spiced Cherry Wine

This makes a good holiday drink or is a pleasing, warming beverage on a chilly evening. The black cherry juice provides anti-inflammatory flavonoids, and the cinnamon and ginger help reduce blood fats and sugars.

2	4-inch (10 cm) cinnamon sticks	2
2	star anise pods	2
2 tsp	minced fresh gingerroot	10 mL
3 cups	unsweetened black cherry juice	750 mL
1 cup	red wine	250 mL
2 tsp	inositol powder	10 mL
½ cup	prickly pear juice	125 mL

1. In a saucepan, combine cinnamon sticks, star anise, ginger, cherry juice and wine. Place over low heat, cover and bring to a simmer (this will take about 20 minutes).

2. Strain through a fine-mesh sieve and discard spices. Stir in inositol powder and prickly pear juice. Pour into mugs and serve warm.

Carrot Pineapple Ginger Breakfast Blend

	Makes 2 to 3 servings	

Carrots, pineapples and ginger are fabulous together, and very nourishing. The addition of flaxseed oil, prickly pear juice, brewer's yeast, inositol and lecithin boost the medicinal value.

Tip

Store any leftover juice in the blender jug in the refrigerator. Blend again before serving and use within the day.

• Blender

4	rosemary leaves	4
1 tbsp	chopped fresh gingerroot	15 mL
2 tsp	lecithin granules or liquid	10 mL
2 tsp	inositol powder	10 mL
1 tsp	brewer's yeast	5 mL
	Grated zest of 1 orange	
1 cup	freshly squeezed orange juice	250 mL
1 tbsp	flaxseed oil	15 mL
3 cups	carrot juice	750 mL
2 cups	unsweetened pineapple juice	500 mL
¼ to	prickly pear juice	60 to
½ cup		125 mL
	Fresh fruit pieces or chunks (grapes or pineapple or apple chunks)	
	Rosemary sprigs	

1. In blender, combine rosemary leaves, ginger, lecithin, inositol powder, brewer's yeast, orange zest, orange juice and flaxseed oil; purée until smooth. Add carrot juice, pineapple juice and prickly pear juice to taste; blend until incorporated.

2. Skewer a piece of fruit on each rosemary sprig. Pour juice into glasses and garnish with rosemary.

Blueberry Smoothie

Makes 2 servings

Blueberries are high in flavonoids, and soy milk offers hormone- and blood sugar–balancing effects. The addition of the nutritional agents improves the medicinal value of this delicious, nutritious drink.

- **Blender**

1 cup	blueberries	250 mL
1 tsp	inositol powder	5 mL
1 tsp	lecithin granules or liquid	5 mL
½ tsp	brewer's yeast	2 mL
3 cups	plain soy milk	750 mL
2 tbsp	prickly pear juice	30 mL
1 tbsp	flaxseed oil	15 mL

1. In blender, combine blueberries, inositol powder, lecithin, brewer's yeast, soy milk, prickly pear juice and flaxseed oil; purée until smooth.

2. Pour into glasses and serve cold.

Maca Mango Smoothie

Makes 2 servings

Ripe mangos are absolutely heavenly — so sweet and delicious that this smoothie satisfies any sugar or dessert craving. Maca has numerous hormone-balancing and circulation-enhancing effects.

Tip
Store any leftover smoothie in the blender jug in the refrigerator. Blend again before serving and use within the day.

- **Blender**

1	mango, chopped	1
2 tbsp	maca powder	30 mL
1 tsp	lecithin granules or liquid	5 mL
½ tsp	brewer's yeast	2 mL
3 cups	plain almond milk	750 mL
1 tbsp	cod liver oil	15 mL

1. In blender, combine mango, maca powder, lecithin, brewer's yeast, almond milk and cod liver oil; purée until smooth.

2. Pour into glasses and serve cold.

Raspberry Hibiscus Smoothie

Makes 2 to 3 servings

This beautiful pink smoothie is satisfying, filling and loaded with valuable nutrients.

Tip

Because cod liver oil has a strong flavor of both liver and fish, most commercial products use fruit flavors to improve its palatability. Lemon-flavored cod liver oil is one of the most popular, and is readily available.

- **Blender**

1 cup	fresh or frozen raspberries	250 mL
1/4 cup	maca powder	60 mL
1 tsp	lecithin granules or liquid	5 mL
1/2 tsp	brewer's yeast	2 mL
3 cups	plain soy milk, chilled	750 mL
1 cup	hibiscus tea, chilled (see tip, page 249)	250 mL
1 tbsp	lemon-flavored cod liver oil	15 mL
1 tsp	agave nectar	5 mL
2	drops vitamin D3 liquid (see tip, page 265)	2

1. In blender, combine raspberries, maca powder, lecithin, brewer's yeast, soy milk, hibiscus tea, cod liver oil, agave nectar and vitamin D3; purée until smooth.

2. Pour into glasses and serve cold.

Almond Butter Smoothie

Makes 2 servings

This rich and satisfying smoothie makes a great breakfast.

Tip

Store any leftover smoothie in the blender jug in the refrigerator. Blend again before serving and use within the day.

- **Blender**

1 tsp	inositol powder	5 mL
1 tsp	lecithin granules or liquid	5 mL
1/2 tsp	brewer's yeast	2 mL
4 cups	plain soy milk	1 L
1/2 cup	natural almond butter	125 mL
1 tbsp	flaxseed oil	15 mL

1. In blender, combine inositol powder, lecithin, brewer's yeast, soy milk, almond butter and flaxseed oil; purée until smooth.

2. Pour into glasses and serve cold.

Banana Walnut Smoothie

Makes 2 servings

Walnuts are high in vitamin E and omega-3 fatty acids, and the milk and banana make a good base.

Tip

Store any leftover smoothie in the blender jug in the refrigerator. Blend again before serving and use within the day.

Variation

Substitute Stevia Tea (page 254) for the apple juice.

- **Blender**

4 to 5	walnut halves	4 to 5
½	banana, cut into chunks	½
2 tsp	lecithin granules or liquid	10 mL
1 tsp	inositol powder	5 mL
3 cups	plain soy milk or other dairy or non-dairy milk	750 mL
½ cup	unsweetened apple, pear or other fruit juice, chilled	125 mL
2 tsp	walnut oil or other nut oil	10 mL
2	drops vitamin D3 liquid (see tip, page 265)	2

1. In blender, combine walnut halves to taste, banana, lecithin, inositol powder, soy milk, apple juice, walnut oil and vitamin D3; purée until smooth.

2. Pour into glasses and serve cold.

Coffee Carob Smoothie

Makes 2 servings

Carob powder is a rich source of *D-chiro-inositol*, and the addition of the other medicinal ingredients makes this smoothie healthy and nourishing.

Tip

Store any leftover smoothie in the blender jug in the refrigerator. Blend again before serving and use within the day.

- **Blender**

½	banana, cut into chunks	½
2 tsp	carob powder	10 mL
1 to 2 tsp	finely ground coffee	5 to 10 mL
1 tsp	lecithin granules or liquid	5 mL
½ tsp	brewer's yeast	2 mL
2 cups	plain soy milk, chilled	500 mL
1 cup	nonfat plain yogurt	250 mL
2 tsp	flaxseed oil	10 mL
2	drops vitamin D3 liquid (see tip, page 265)	2
	Cocoa nibs	

1. In blender, combine banana, carob powder, coffee to taste, lecithin, brewer's yeast, soy milk, yogurt, flaxseed oil and vitamin D3; purée until smooth.

2. Pour into glasses and garnish each with 1 tsp (5 mL) cocoa nibs. Serve cold.

Piña Macolada

Maca powder has a pleasant flavor and a fine texture that's easy to work into smoothies. Pineapple has anti-inflammatory effects and is purported to support weight-loss efforts.

Tips

Vitamin D plays an important role in insulin reception and blood sugar regulation. Liquid vitamin D supplements, available at health food stores, typically supply 1,000 IUs per drop.

Store any leftover smoothie in the blender jug in the refrigerator. Blend again before serving and use within the day.

- **Blender**

2 cups	chopped fresh pineapple	500 mL
1 tbsp	unsweetened coconut flakes	15 mL
1 tbsp	maca powder	15 mL
2 tsp	lecithin granules	10 mL
1 tsp	inositol powder	5 mL
½ tsp	brewer's yeast	2 mL
2 cups	pineapple-coconut juice or unsweetened pineapple juice, chilled	500 mL
1 cup	nonfat plain yogurt	250 mL
½ cup	coconut milk	125 ml
1 tbsp	flaxseed oil	15 mL
2	drops vitamin D3 liquid (see tip, at left)	2

1. Spread pineapple in a single layer on a baking sheet or dish. Freeze for 1 to 2 hours or until semi-frozen.

2. In blender, combine semi-frozen pineapple, coconut flakes, maca powder, lecithin, inositol powder, brewer's yeast, pineapple-coconut juice, yogurt, coconut milk, flaxseed oil and vitamin D3; purée until smooth.

3. Pour into glasses and serve cold.

Pineapple Coconut Maca Flax Smoothie

Makes 2 servings

The classic tropical combination of pineapple and coconut makes a creamy base for the medicinal ingredients in this smoothie.

- **Blender**

1 tbsp	maca powder	15 mL
1 tsp	ground flax seeds (flaxseed meal)	5 mL
3 cups	unsweetened pineapple juice	750 mL
½ cup	coconut milk	125 mL
1 tsp	lecithin granules or liquid	5 mL
2	drops vitamin D3 liquid (see tip, page 265)	2

1. In blender, combine maca powder, flax seeds, pineapple juice, coconut milk, lecithin and vitamin D3; purée until smooth.

2. Pour into glasses and serve cold.

Icy Banana Cashew Smoothie

Makes 2 servings

This smoothie makes a great summer breakfast or ice cream substitute. Loaded with medicinal ingredients, it's satisfying and filling enough to be meal in and of itself.

- **Blender**

1	ripe banana, cut into chunks	1
¼ cup	raw cashews	60 mL
2 tbsp	whey powder	30 mL
2 tbsp	maca powder	30 mL
1 tsp	inositol powder	5 mL
3 cups	plain rice milk	750 mL
¼ cup	prickly pear juice	60 mL
2 tsp	flaxseed oil	10 mL
1 cup	ice cubes	250 mL

1. In blender, combine banana, cashews, whey powder, maca powder, inositol powder, rice milk, prickly pear juice and flaxseed oil; purée until smooth. Add ice cubes and blend slightly.

2. Pour into glasses and serve cold (within the hour).

Banana Mango Hibiscus Smoothie

Keep some frozen bananas on hand to whip up this healthy treat, which is filling enough to serve as a breakfast.

Tips

To avoid wasting bananas that are reaching perfection before you can eat them, peel the bananas and cut them into bite-size pieces. Freeze the pieces on a paper plate or other freezer-safe plate. Freeze for about 4 hours or until solid. Transfer to a freezer bag and freeze to use over the next several weeks when making smoothies.

Store any leftover smoothie in the blender jug in the refrigerator. Blend again before serving and use within the day.

● **Blender**

1 cup	frozen banana pieces (see tip, at left)	250 mL
1	small mango, chopped	1
1 tsp	finely chopped fresh gingerroot	5 mL
1 tbsp	raw cashews	15 mL
2 tsp	lecithin granules or liquid	10 mL
½ cup	hibiscus tea, chilled (see tip, page 249)	125 mL
¼ cup	prickly pear juice	60 mL
¼ to ½ cup	unsweetened fruit juice (optional)	60 to 125 mL

1. Let bananas thaw for about 15 minutes, until slightly softened.

2. In blender, combine banana, mango, ginger, cashews, lecithin, hibiscus tea and prickly pear juice; purée until smooth. Add fruit juice to thin, if desired.

3. Pour into glasses and serve cold.

Raspberry Yogurt Smoothie

Makes 2 servings

Raspberries are abundant in the early summer — and in the freezer section of most groceries year-round.

Tip

Store any leftover smoothie in the blender jug in the refrigerator. Blend again before serving and use within the day.

- **Blender**

1 cup	fresh or frozen raspberries	250 mL
1 tbsp	maca powder	15 mL
1 tsp	inositol powder	5 mL
1 tsp	brewer's yeast	5 mL
1 cup	nonfat plain yogurt	250 mL
1 cup	plain soy milk, chilled	250 mL
2	drops vitamin D3 liquid (see tip, page 265)	2

1. In blender, combine raspberries, maca powder, inositol powder, brewer's yeast, yogurt, soy milk and vitamin D3; purée until smooth.

2. Pour into glasses and serve cold.

Rose Essence Nectar

Makes 4 servings

This unusual, delightful, delicately flavored drink is very cooling on a hot summer day.

Tips

To crush ice cubes, place them inside a kitchen towel and pound them with a hammer.

Rose water is available in gourmet shops, Middle Eastern food stores and herb shops.

- **Blender**

4 cups	nonfat or low-fat plain yogurt	1 L
2 cups	crushed ice	500 mL
2 cups	sparkling mineral water	500 mL
½ cup	Stevia Tea (page 254), chilled	125 mL
2 tbsp	rose water	30 mL
	Red or pink rose petals (optional)	

1. In blender, combine yogurt, ice, mineral water, stevia tea and rose water; blend briefly, being sure to leave the ice a bit chunky (it is best to blend in short bursts on a low setting, to prevent the mineral water from frothing up).

2. If desired, place 4 or 5 rose petals in each glass. Pour in yogurt mixture. Stir once with a long-handled spoon and serve immediately.

Cucumber Slushie

Don't overlook vegetables as a base for refreshing beverages.

Tip

Store any leftover slush in the blender jug in the refrigerator. Blend again before serving and use within the day.

● **Blender**

2	large cucumbers, peeled and coarsely chopped	2
2 tsp	fresh rosemary leaves	10 mL
1 tsp	dulse flakes (optional)	5 mL
2 cups	cold spring water	500 mL
	Grated zest of 1 lemon	
½ cup	freshly squeezed lemon juice	125 mL
2 tbsp	agave nectar	30 mL
	Rosemary sprigs	

1. In blender, combine cucumber, rosemary leaves, dulse flakes (if using), water, lemon zest, lemon juice and agave nectar; purée until smooth.

2. Pour into glasses and serve cold, garnished with rosemary sprigs.

Watermelon Slush

This delicious slush is low in calories, easy to prepare and makes an effective dieter's drink.

● **Blender**

2 cups	chunks watermelon	500 mL
6	large ice cubes	6
1 tsp	inositol powder	5 mL
	Grated zest of 1 lemon	
½ cup	freshly squeezed lemon juice	125 mL
¼ cup	prickly pear juice	60 mL
2 tbsp	Stevia Tea (page 254), chilled	30 mL

1. In blender, combine watermelon, ice cubes, inositol powder, lemon zest, lemon juice, prickly pear juice and stevia tea; purée until slushy.

2. Pour into glasses and serve immediately.

Red Grape Slush

Prickly pear juice and grapes make a fantastic combination, and the inositol powder adds medicinal value.

Tip

Dried hibiscus flowers are available in herb shops and health food stores. If you can't find them, use 2 commercial tea bags that have hibiscus as a main ingredient.

- **Blender**

1 tbsp	dried hibiscus flowers (see tip, at left)	15 mL
1 cup	boiling water	250 mL
1 tsp	inositol powder	10 mL
2 tsp	agave nectar	10 mL
2 cups	seedless red grapes	500 mL
2 cups	sparkling mineral water	500 mL
1/4 cup	prickly pear juice	60 mL

1. Place hibiscus flowers in a teapot or saucepan. Pour in boiling water, cover and let steep for 10 to 15 minutes. Strain through a tea strainer or fine-mesh sieve into a container. Stir in inositol powder and agave nectar until dissolved. Cover and refrigerate for 4 hours, until chilled, or for up to 2 days.

2. In blender, combine chilled tea and grapes; purée until smooth. Transfer to a pitcher and stir in mineral water and prickly pear juice. Pour into glasses and serve immediately.

References

General PCOS References, Prevalence, Definition, Symptoms

Balen A. Polycystic ovary syndrome and cancer. *Hum Reprod Update*, 2001;7(6):522–25.

Burzawa JK, Schmeler KM, Soliman PT, et al. Prospective evaluation of insulin resistance among endometrial cancer patients. *Am J Obstet Gynecol*, 2011 Apr;204(4):355.e1–7.

Carmina E, Lobo R. Polycystic ovary syndrome (PCOS): Arguably the most common endocrinopathy is associated with significant morbidity in women. *J Clin Endocrinol Metab*, 1999 Jun;84(6):1897–99.

Chittenden BG, Fullerton G, Maheshwari A, et al. Polycystic ovary syndrome and the risk of gynaecological cancer: A systematic review. *Reprod Biomed Online*, 2009 Sep;19(3):398–405.

Corbett SJ, McMichael AJ, Prentice AM. Type 2 diabetes, cardiovascular disease, and the evolutionary paradox of the polycystic ovary syndrome: a fertility first hypothesis. *Am J Hum Biol*, 2009 Sep–Oct;21(5):587–98.

Giallauria F, Palomba S, Vigorito C, et al. Androgens in polycystic ovary syndrome: The role of exercise and diet. *Semin Reprod Med*, 2009 Jul;27(4):306–15.

Karkanaki A, Piouka A, Katsikis I, et al. Adiponectin levels reflect the different phenotypes of polycystic ovary syndrome: Study in normal weight, normoinsulinemic patients. *Fertil Steril*, 2009 Aug;92(6):2078–81.

Kulie T, Slattengren A, Redmer J, et al. Obesity and women's health: An evidence-based review. *J Am Board Fam Med*, 2011 Jan–Feb;24(1):75–85.

Shah B, Parnell L, et al. Endometrial thickness, uterine, and ovarian ultrasonographic features in adolescents with polycystic ovarian syndrome. *J Pediatr Adolesc Gynecol*, 2009 Sep;23(3):146–52.

PCOS and Insulin Resistance and Metabolic Syndrome

Alberti KGMM, Zimmet P, Shaw J. Metabolic syndrome — a new world-wide definition. A Consensus Statement from the International Diabetes Federation, 2005 Dec 19.

Badawy A, Elnashar A. Treatment options for polycystic ovary syndrome. *Int J Women's Health*, 2011 Feb 8; 3:25–35.

Corbett SJ, McMichael AJ, Prentice AM. Type 2 diabetes, cardiovascular disease, and the evolutionary paradox of the polycystic ovary syndrome: A fertility first hypothesis. *Am J Hum Biol*, 2009 Sep–Oct;21(5):587–98.

Dahlgren E, Janson P, Johansson S, et al. Polycystic ovary syndrome and risk for myocardial infarction: Evaluated from a risk factor model based on a prospective population study of women. *Acta Obstet Gynecol Scand*, 1992 Dec;71(8):599–604.

Ford E, Giles W, Dietz W. Prevalence of the metabolic syndrome among US adults: Findings from the third National Health and Nutrition Examination Survey. *JAMA*, 2002 Jan 16;287(3):356–59.

Ghatta S, Ramarao P. Increased contractile responses to 5-hydroxytryptamine and angiotensin II in high fat diet fed rat thoracic aorta. *Lipids Health Dis*, 2004 Aug 2;3(1):19.

Halperin IJ, Kumar SS, Stroup DF, et al. The association between the combined oral contraceptive pill and insulin resistance, dysglycemia and dyslipidemia in women with polycystic ovary syndrome: A systematic review and meta-analysis of observational studies. *Hum Reprod*, 2011 Jan;26(1):191–201.

Hirschberg AL. Polycystic ovary syndrome, obesity and reproductive implications. *Women's Health* (Lond Engl), 2009 Sep;5(5):529–40.

Kilic S, Yilmaz N, Zulfikaroglu E, et al. Inflammatory-metabolic parameters in obese and nonobese normoandrogenemic polycystic ovary syndrome during metformin and oral contraceptive treatment. *Gynecol Endocrinol*, 2011 Sep;27(9):622–29.

Macías-Robles MD, Maciá-Bobes C, Yano-Escudero R, et al. Metformin-induced lactic acidosis due to acute renal failure. *An Sist Sanit Navar*, 2011 Jan–Apr;34(1):115–18.

Miatello R, Cruzado M, Risler N. Mechanisms of cardiovascular changes in an experimental model of syndrome X and pharmacological intervention on the renin-angiotensin-system. *Curr Vasc Pharmacol*, 2004 Oct;2(4):371–77.

Moran LJ, Meyer C, Hutchison SK, et al. Novel inflammatory markers in overweight women with and without polycystic ovary syndrome and following pharmacological intervention. *J Endocrinol Invest*, 2009 Dec;32(11):873–76.

Motta AB. Mechanisms involved in metformin action in the treatment of polycystic ovary syndrome. *Curr Pharm Des*, 2009;15(26):3074–77.

Oh JY, Sung YA, Lee HJ, et al. Optimal waist circumference for prediction of metabolic syndrome in young Korean women with polycystic ovary syndrome. *Obesity* (Silver Spring), 2010 Mar;18(3):593–97.

Ornstein RM, Copperman NM, Jacobson MS. Effect of weight loss on menstrual function in adolescents with polycystic ovary syndrome. *J Pediatr Adolesc Gynecol*, 2011 Jun;24(3):161–65.

Otta CF, Wior M, Iraci GS, et al. Clinical, metabolic, and endocrine parameters in response to metformin and lifestyle intervention in women with polycystic ovary syndrome: A randomized, double-blind, and placebo control trial. *Gynecol Endocrinol*, 2010 Mar;26(3):173–78.

Panza F, Frisardi V, Seripa D, et al. Metabolic syndrome, mild cognitive impairment, and dementia. *Curr Alzheimer Res*, 2011 Aug;8(5):492–509.

Poitout V, Robertson RP. Glucolipotoxicity: Fuel excess and beta-cell dysfunction. *Endocr Rev*, 2008 May;29(3):351–66.

Roberts CK, Liang K, Barnard RJ, et al. HMG-CoA reductase, cholesterol 7alpha-hydroxylase, LDL receptor, SR-B1, and ACAT in diet-induced syndrome X. *Kidney Int*, 2004 Oct;66(4):1503–11.

Rocha MP, Maranhão RC, Seydell TM, et al. Metabolism of triglyceride-rich lipoproteins and lipid transfer to high-density lipoprotein in young obese and normal-weight patients with polycystic ovary syndrome. *Fertil Steril*, 2010 Apr;93(6):1948–56.

Samy N, Hashim M, Sayed M, et al. Clinical significance of inflammatory markers in polycystic ovary syndrome: Their relationship to insulin resistance and body mass index. *Dis Markers*, 2009;26(4):163–70.

Seneviratne H, Lankeshwara D, Wijeratne S, et al. Serum insulin patterns and the relationship between insulin sensitivity and glycaemic profile in women with polycystic ovary syndrome. *BJOG*, Dec;116(13):1722–28.

Sharkey D, Symonds M, Budge H. Adipose tissue inflammation: Developmental ontogeny and consequences of gestational nutrient restriction in offspring. *Endocrinology*, 2009 Aug;150(8):3913–20.

Svendsen P, Madsbad S, Nilas L, et al. Expression of 11beta-hydroxysteroid dehydrogenase 1 and 2 in subcutaneous adipose tissue of lean and obese women with and without polycystic ovary syndrome. *Int J Obes* (Lond), 2009 Nov;33(11):1249–56.

Ten S, Maclaren N. Insulin resistance syndrome in children. *J Clin Endocrinol Metab*, 2004 Jun;89(6):2526–39.

Thomas T, Pfeiffer A. Foods for the prevention of diabetes: How do they work? *Diabetes Metab Res Rev*, 2012 Jan;28(1):25–49.

Verhaeghe J. Hormonal contraception in women with the metabolic syndrome: A narrative review. *Eur J Contracept Reprod Health Care*, 2010 Oct; 15(5):305–13.

Verit FF. High sensitive serum C-reactive protein and its relationship with other cardiovascular risk factors in normoinsulinemic polycystic ovary patients without metabolic syndrome. *Arch Gynecol Obstet*, 2010 Jun; 281(6):1009–14.

World Health Organization. *Diabetes*. Fact sheet no. 312, 2001 Aug. Available at: http://www.who.int/mediacentre/factsheets/fs312/en/.

PCOS and Fertility

Alshammari A, Hanley A, Ni A, et al. Does the presence of polycystic ovary syndrome increase the risk of obstetrical complications in women with gestational diabetes? *J Maternal Fetal Neonatal Med*, 2009 Aug;27:1–5.

Bausenwein J, Serke H, Eberle K, et al. Elevated levels of oxidised low-density lipoprotein and of catalase activity in follicular fluid of obese women. *Mol Hum Reprod*, 2010 Feb;16(2):117–24.

Carmichael AR. Can *Vitex agnus-castus* be used for the treatment of mastalgia? What is the current evidence? *Evid Based Complement Alternat Med*, 2008 Sep;5(3):247–50.

Ciotta L, Stracquadanio M, Pagano I, et al. Effects of myo-inositol supplementation on oocyte's quality in PCOS patients: A double blind trial. *Eur Rev Med Pharmacol Sci*, 2011 May;15(5):509–14.

Döll M. The premenstrual syndrome: effectiveness of *Vitex agnus-castus*. *Med Monatsschr Pharm*, 2009 May;32(5):186–91.

Fulghesu AM, Ciampelli M, Muzj G, et al. N-acetyl-cysteine treatment improves insulin sensitivity in women with polycystic ovary syndrome. *Fertil Steril*, 2002 Jun;77(6):1128–35.

Hirschberg AL. Polycystic ovary syndrome, obesity and reproductive implications. *Women's Health* (Lond Engl), 2009 Sep;5(5):529–40.

Hu Y, Xin HL, Zhang QY, et al. Anti-nociceptive and anti-hyperprolactinemia activities of *Fructus viticis* and its effective fractions and chemical constituents. *Phytomedicine*, 2007 Oct;14(10):668–74.

Hughes E, Brown J, Collins JJ, et al. Clomiphene citrate for unexplained subfertility in women. *Cochrane Database Syst Rev*, 2010 Jan 20;(1):CD000057.

Ibrahim NA, Shalaby AS, Farag RS, et al. Gynecological efficacy and chemical investigation of *Vitex agnus-castus* L. fruits growing in Egypt. *Nat Prod Res*, 2008 Apr 15;22(6):537–46.

Kostrzak A, Warenik-Szymankiewicz A, Meczekalski B. The role of serum PRL bioactivity evaluation in hyperprolactinaemic women with different menstrual disorders. *Gynecol Endocrinol*, 2009 Dec;25(12):799–806.

Lam P, Johnson I, Raine-Fenning N. Endometrial blood flow is impaired in women with polycystic ovarian syndrome who are clinically hyperandrogenic. *Ultrasound Obstet Gynecol*, 2009 Sep;34(3):326–34.

Milewicz A, Gejdel E, Sworen H, et al. *Vitex agnus castus* extract in the treatment of luteal phase defects due to latent hyperprolactinemia: Results of a randomized placebo-controlled double-blind study. *Arzneimittelforschung*, 1993 Jul;43(7):752–6.

Nasr A. Effect of N-acetyl-cysteine after ovarian drilling in clomiphene citrate-resistant PCOS women: A pilot study. *Reprod Biomed Online*, 2010 Mar;20(3):403–9.

Ott J, Aust S, Kurz C, et al. Elevated antithyroid peroxidase antibodies indicating Hashimoto's thyroiditis are associated with the treatment response in infertile women with polycystic ovary syndrome. *Fertil Steril*, 2010 Dec;94(7):2895–97.

Palomba S, Falbo A, Zullo F. Management strategies for ovulation induction in women with polycystic ovary syndrome and known clomifene citrate resistance. *Curr Opin Obstet Gynecol*, 2009 Dec;21(6):465–73.

Papaleo E, Unfer V, Baillargeon JP, et al. Contribution of myo-inositol to reproduction. *Eur J Obstet Gynecol Reprod Biol*, 2009 Dec;147(2):120–23.

Qian X, Yu H. Effects of shenghua decoction on hemorheology, thrombosis and microcirculation. *Zhongguo Zhong Yao Za Zhi*, 2011 Feb;36(4):514–18.

Qublan HS, Al-Khaderei S, Abu-Salem AN, et al. Metformin in the treatment of clomiphene citrate-resistant women with polycystic ovary syndrome undergoing in vitro fertilisation treatment: A randomised controlled trial. *J Obstet Gynaecol*, 2009 Oct;29(7):651–55.

Racho? D, Teede H. Ovarian function and obesity — interrelationship, impact on women's reproductive lifespan and treatment options. *Mol Cell Endocrinal*, 2010 Mar 25;316(2):172–79.

Rizk AY, Bedaiwy MA, A l-Inany HG. N-acetyl-cysteine is a novel adjuvant to clomiphene citrate in clomiphene citrate-resistant patients with polycystic ovary syndrome. *Fertil Steril*, 2005 Feb;83(2):367–70.

Sartorelli DS, Franco LJ, Gimeno SG, et al. Dietary fructose, fruits, fruit juices and glucose tolerance status in Japanese-Brazilians. *Nutr Metab Cardiovasc Dis*, 2009 Feb;19(2):77–83.

Tosi F, Dorizzi R, Castello R, et al. Body fat and insulin resistance independently predict increased serum C-reactive protein in hyperandrogenic women with polycystic ovary syndrome. *Eur J Endocrinol*, 2009 Nov;161(5):737–45.

Trokoudes KM, Skordis N, Picolos MK. Infertility and thyroid disorders. *Curr Opin Obstet Gynecol*, 2006 Aug;18(4):446–51.

Vlahos NF, Economopoulos KP, Fotiou S. Endometriosis, in vitro fertilisation and the risk of gynaecological malignancies, including ovarian and breast cancer. *Best Pract Res Clin Obstet Gynaecol*, 2010 Feb;24(1):39–50.

Wilkes S, Murdoch A. Obesity and female fertility: A primary care perspective. *J Fam Plann Reprod Health Care*, 2009 Jul;35(3):181–85.

Xia YW, Cai LX, Zhang SC. Therapeutic effect of Chinese herbal medicines for nourishing blood and reinforcing shen in treating patients with anovulatory sterility of shen-deficiency type and its influence on the hemodynamics in ovarian and uterine arteries. *Zhongguo Zhong Xi Yi Jie He Za Zhi*, 2004 Apr;24(4):299–302.

Ye Q, Zhang Qy, Zheng Cj, et al. Casticin, a flavonoid isolated from *Vitex rotundifolia*, inhibits prolactin release in vivo and in vitro. *Acta Pharmacol Sin*, 2010 Dec;31(12):1564–68.

PCOS and Thyroid Function

Abalovich M, Llesuy S, Gutierrez S, et al. Peripheral parameters of oxidative stress in Graves' disease: The effects of methimazole and 131 iodine treatments. *Clin Endocrinol* (Oxf), 2003 Sep;59(3):321–27.

Anaforoglu I, Topbas M, Algun E. Relative associations of polycystic ovarian syndrome versus metabolic syndrome with thyroid function: Volume, nodularity and autoimmunity. *J Endocrinol Invest*, 2011 Oct; 34(9):e259–64.

Dittrich R, Beckmann M, Oppelt P, et al. Thyroid hormone receptors and reproduction. *J Reprod Immunol*, 2011 Jun;90(1):58–66.

Dittrich R, Kajaia N, Cupisti S, et al. Association of thyroid-stimulating hormone with insulin resistance and androgen parameters in women with PCOS. *Reprod Biomed Online*, 2009 Sep;19(3):319–25.

Donnini D, Ambesi-Impiombato F, Curcio F. Thyrotropin stimulates production of procoagulant and vasodilative factors in human aortic endothelial cells. *Thyroid*, 2003 Jun;13(6):517–21.

Ganie MA, Marwaha RK, Aggarwal R, et al. High prevalence of polycystic ovary syndrome characteristics in girls with euthyroid chronic lymphocytic thyroiditis: A case-control study. *Eur J Endocrinol*, 2010 Jun;162(6):1117–22.

Gleicher N, Barad D, Weghofer A. Functional autoantibodies: A new paradigm in autoimmunity? *Autoimmune Rev*, 2007 Nov;7(1):42–45.

Janssen OE, Mehlmauer N, Hahn S, et al. High prevalence of autoimmune thyroiditis in patients with polycystic ovary syndrome. *Eur J Endocrinol*, 2004 Mar;150(3):363–69.

Krassas GE, Poppe K, Glinoer D. Thyroid function and human reproductive health. *Endocr Rev*, 2010 Oct;31(5):702–55.

Lamberg BA. Endemic goiter — iodine deficiency disorders. *Ann Med*, 1991 Oct;23(4):367–72.

Lightowler H, Davies G. Iodine intake and iodine deficiency in vegans as assessed by the duplicate-portion technique and urinary iodine excretion. *Br J Nutr*, 1998 Dec;80(6):529–35.

Mardarowicz G, Lopatynski J, Nicer T. Metabolic syndrome. *Ann Univ Mariae Curie Sklodowska Med*, 2003;58(1):426-31.

Mohamadin A, Hammad L, El-Bab M, et al. Attenuation of oxidative stress in plasma and tissues of rats with experimentally induced hyperthyroidism by caffeic acid phenylethyl ester. *Basic Clin Pharmacol Toxicol*, 2007 Feb;100(2):84–90.

Monzani F, Dardano A, Caraccio N. Does treating subclinical hypothyroidism improve markers of cardiovascular risk? *Treat Endocrinol*, 2006;5(2):65–81.

Morteza Taghavi S, Rokni H, Fatemi S. Metformin decreases thyrotropin in overweight women with polycystic ovarian syndrome and hypothyroidism. *Diab Vasc Dis Res*, 2011 Jan;8(1):47–48.

Muderris II, Boztosun A, Oner G. Effect of thyroid hormone replacement therapy on ovarian volume and androgen hormones in patients with untreated primary hypothyroidism. *F Ann Saudi Med*, 2011 Mar–Apr;31(2):145–51.

Mueller A, Schöfl C, Dittrich R, et al. Thyroid-stimulating hormone is associated with insulin resistance independently of body mass index and age in women with polycystic ovary syndrome. *Hum Reprod*, 2009 Nov;24(11):2924–30.

Nohr L, Rasmussen LB, Straand J. Resin from the mukul myrrh tree, guggul: Can it be used for treating hypercholesterolemia? A randomized, controlled study. *Complement Ther Med*, 2009 Jan;17(1):16–22.

Ott J, Aust S, Kurz C, et al. Elevated antithyroid peroxidase antibodies indicating Hashimoto's thyroiditis are associated with the treatment response in infertile women with polycystic ovary syndrome. *Fertil Steril*, 2010 Dec;94(7):2895–97.

Panda S, Kar A. Guggulu (*Commiphora mukul*) potentially ameliorates hypothyroidism in female mice. *Phytother Res*, 2005 Jan;19(1):78–80.

Panda S, Kar A. Gugulu (*Commiphora mukul*) induces triiodothyronine production: Possible involvement of lipid peroxidation. *Life Sci*, 1999;65(12):PL137–41.

Panico A, Lupoli GA, Fonderico F, et al. Multiple ovarian cysts in a young girl with severe hypothyroidism. *Thyroid*, 2007 Dec;17(12):1289–93.

Poppe K, Velkeniers B, Glinoer D. Thyroid disease and female reproduction. *Clin Endocrinol* (Oxf), 2007 Mar;66(3):309–21.

Reismann P, Somogyi A. Diabetes and thyroid disorders. *Orv Hetil*, 2011 Mar 27;152(13):516–19.

Rotondi M, Cappelli C, Magri F, et al. Thyroidal effect of metformin treatment in patients with polycystic ovary syndrome. *Clin Endocrinol* (Oxf), 2011 Sep; 75(3):378–81.

Smyth P. The thyroid, iodine and breast cancer. *Breast Cancer Res*, 2003;5(5):235–38.

Tripathi Y, Malhotra O, Tripathi S. Thyroid stimulating action of Z-Guggulsterone obtained from *Commiphora mukul*. *Planta Med*, 1984 Feb;50(1):78–80.

Wu J, Xia C, Meier J, et al. The hypolipidemic natural product guggulsterone acts as an antagonist of the bile acid receptor. *Mol Endocrinol*, 2002 Jul;16(7):1590–97.

Herbal, Nutritional and Dietary Therapies for PCOS

Abe M, Ito Y, Oyunzul L, et al. 5alpha-reductase inhibitory activity of free fatty acids contained in saw palmetto extract. *Biol Pharm Bull*, 2009 Apr;32(4):646–50.

Abete I, Goyenechea E, Zulet MA, Martínez JA. Obesity and metabolic syndrome: Potential benefit from specific nutritional components. *Nutr Metab Cardiovasc Dis*, 2011 Sep;21 Suppl 2:B1–15.

Adolphe JL, Whiting SJ, Juurlink BH, et al. Health effects with consumption of the flax lignan secoisolariciresinol diglucoside. *Br J Nutr*, 2010 Apr;103(7):929–38.

Alarcon-Aguilar FJ, Valdes-Arzate A, Xolalpa-Molina S, et al. Hypoglycemic activity of two polysaccharides isolated from *Opuntia ficus-indica* and *O. streptacantha*. *Proc West Pharmacol Soc*, 2003;46:139–42.

Armanini D, Castello R, Scaroni C, et al. Treatment of polycystic ovary syndrome with spironolactone plus licorice. *Eur J Obstet Gynecol Reprod Biol*, 2007 Mar;131(1):61–67.

Armanini D, Mattarello MJ, Fiore C, et al. Licorice reduces serum testosterone in healthy women. *Steroids*, 2004 Oct–Nov;69(11–12):763–6.

Ayami Matsushima, Xiaohui Liu, Hiroyuki Okada, et al. Bisphenol AF is a full agonist for the estrogen receptor ER? but a highly specific antagonist for ER?. *Environ Health Perspect*, 2010 September;118(9):1267–72.

Babey S, Jones M, Yu H, et al. Bubbling over: Soda consumption and its link to obesity in California. *Policy Brief UCLA Cent Health Policy Res*, 2009 Sep;(PB2009-5):1–8.

Bai HY, Zou WJ, Gao XP. Influence of *Pueraria thomsonii* on insulin resistance induced by dexamethasone. *Zhongguo Zhong Yao Za Zhi*, 2004 Apr;29(4):356–58.

Baillargeon JP, Nestler JE, Ostlund RE, et al. Greek hyperinsulinemic women, with or without polycystic ovary syndrome, display altered inositols metabolism. *Hum Reprod*, 2008 Jun;23(6):1439–46.

Baños G, Pérez-Torres I, El Hafidi M. Medicinal agents in the metabolic syndrome. *Cardiovasc Hematol Agents Med Chem*, 2008 Oct;6(4):237–52.

Baquer NZ, Kumar P, Taha A, et al. Metabolic and molecular action of *Trigonella foenum-graecum* (fenugreek) and trace metals in experimental diabetic tissues. *J Biosci*, 2011 Jun;36(2):383–96.

Biden T, Prentki M, Irvine R, et al. Inositol 1,4,5-trisphosphate mobilizes intracellular Ca^{2+} from permeabilized insulin-secreting cells. *Biochem J*, 1984 October 15; 223(2):467–73.

Bonfig W, Gärtner R, Schmidt H. Selenium supplementation does not decrease thyroid peroxidase antibody concentration in children and adolescents with autoimmune thyroiditis. *Scientific World Journal*, 2010 Jun 1;10:990–96.

Boniface R, et al. Pharmacological properties of *Myrtillus anthocyanosides*: Correlation with results of treatment of diabetic microangiopathy. *Study Org Chem*, 1986;23:293–301.

Brahmachari G, Mandal L, Roy R, et al. Stevioside and related compounds — molecules of pharmaceutical promise: A critical overview. *Arch Pharm* (Weinheim), 2011 Jan;344(1):5–19.

Branca F, Lorenzetti S. Health effects of phytoestrogens. *Forum Nutr*, 2005;(57):100–11.

Bretveld R, Thomas C, Scheepers P, et al. Pesticide exposure: The hormonal function of the female reproductive system disrupted? *Reprod Biol Endocrinol*, 2006 May 31;4:30.

Cann SA, van Netten JP, van Netten C. Hypothesis: Iodine, selenium and the development of breast cancer. *Cancer Causes Control*, 2000 Feb;11(2):121–27.

Carlomagno G, Unfer V. Inositol safety: Clinical evidences. *Eur Rev Med Pharmacol Sci*, 2011 Aug; 15(8):931–36.

Cefalu WT, Ye J, Wang ZQ. Efficacy of dietary supplementation with botanicals on carbohydrate metabolism in humans. *Endocr Metab Immune Disord Drug Targets*, 2008 Jun;8(2):78–81.

Chan P, Tomlinson B, Chen YJ, et al. A double-blind placebo-controlled study of the effectiveness and tolerability of oral stevioside in human hypertension. *Br J Clin Pharmacol*, 2000 Sep;50(3):215–20.

Chang J, Wu M, Liu I, et al. Increase of insulin sensitivity by stevioside in fructose-rich chow-fed rats. *Horm Metab Res*, 2005 Oct;37(10):610–16.

Chang S, Liu C, Kuo C, et al. Garlic oil alleviates MAPKs- and IL-6-mediated diabetes-related cardiac hypertrophy in STZ-induced DM rats. *Evid Based Complement Alternat Med*, 2011;2011:950150.

Chao M, Zou D, Zhang Y, et al. Improving insulin resistance with traditional Chinese medicine in type 2 diabetic patients. *Endocrine*, 2009 Oct;36(2):268–74.

Chaturvedula VS, Upreti M, Prakash I. Diterpene glycosides from *Stevia rebaudiana*. *Molecules*, 2011 Apr 28;16(5):3552–62.

Chen T, Chen S, Chan P, et al. Mechanism of the hypoglycemic effect of stevioside, a glycoside of *Stevia rebaudiana*. *Planta Med*, 2005 Feb;71(2):108–13.

Chen Y, Watson H, Gao J, et al. Characterization of the organic component of low-molecular-weight chromium-binding substance and its binding of chromium. *J Nutr*, 2011 Jul;141(7):1225–32.

Choi H, Kim K, Lim CY, et al. Low serum vitamin D is associated with high risk of diabetes in Korean adults. *J Nutr*, 2011 Aug;141(8):1524–28.

Choi M, Lee M, Jung U, et al. Metabolic response of soy pinitol on lipid-lowering, antioxidant and hepatoprotective action in hamsters fed high fat and high cholesterol diet. *Mol Nutr Food Res*, 2009 Jun;53(6):751–59.

Chong MF, Macdonald R, Lovegrove JA. Fruit polyphenols and CVD risk: A review of human intervention studies. *Br J Nutr*, 2010 Oct; 104(Suppl 3):S28–39.

Christ S. *List of Foods High in D-Chiro-Inositol*. Available at: http://www.ehow.com/list_5960312_list-foods-high-d_chiro_inositol.html#ixzz1Vtqafn3Y.

Cornish SM, Chilibeck PD, Paus-Jennsen L, et al. A randomized controlled trial of the effects of flaxseed lignan complex on metabolic syndrome composite score and bone mineral in older adults. *Appl Physiol Nutr Metab*, 2009 Apr;34(2):89–98.

Costantino D, Minozzi G, Minozzi E, et al. Metabolic and hormonal effects of myo-inositol in women with polycystic ovary syndrome: A double-blind trial. *Eur Rev Med Pharmacol Sci*, 2009 Mar–Apr; 13(2):105–10.

Davies DM, Holdsworth ES, Sherriff JL. The isolation of glucose tolerance factors from brewer's yeast and their relationship to chromium. *Biochem Med*, 1985 Jun;33(3):297–311.

de Lordes Lima M, Cruz T, Pousada JC, et al. The effect of magnesium supplementation in increasing doses on the control of type 2 diabetes. *Diabetes Care*, 1998 May;21(5):682–86.

Dey D, Pal BC, Biswas T, et al. A lupinoside prevented fatty acid induced inhibition of insulin sensitivity in 3T3 L1 adipocytes. *Mol Cell Biochem*, 2007 Jun; 300(1–2):149–57.

Diwakar BT, Dutta PK, Lokesh BR, et al. Bio-availability and metabolism of n-3 fatty acid rich garden cress (*Lepidium sativum*) seed oil in albino rats. *Prostaglandins Leukot Essent Fatty Acids*, 2008 Feb; 78(2):123–30.

Dodin S, Cunnane SC, Mâsse B, et al. Flaxseed on cardiovascular disease markers in healthy menopausal women: A randomized, double-blind, placebo-controlled trial. *Nutrition*, 2008 Jan;24(1):23–30.

Dubois L, Farmer A, Girard M, et al. Regular sugar-sweetened beverage consumption between meals increases risk of overweight among preschool-aged children. *J Am Diet Assoc*, 2007 Jun;107(6):924–34.

Dyrskog SE, Jeppesen PB, Colombo M, et al. Preventive effects of a soy-based diet supplemented with stevioside on the development of the metabolic syndrome and type 2 diabetes in Zucker diabetic fatty rats. *Metabolism*, 2005 Sep;54(9):1181–88.

Eddouks M, Maghrani M. Effect of *Lepidium sativum* L. on renal glucose reabsorption and urinary TGF-beta 1 levels in diabetic rats. *Phytother Res*, 2008 Jan;22(1):1–5.

Eddouks M, Maghrani M, Zeggwagh NA, et al. Study of the hypoglycaemic activity of *Lepidium sativum* L. aqueous extract in normal and diabetic rats. *J Ethnopharmacol*, 2005 Feb 28;97(2):391–95.

el-Sheikh MM, Dakkak MR, Saddique A. The effect of Permixon on androgen receptors. *Acta Obstet Gynecol Scand*, 1988;67(5):397–99.

Ennouri M, Fetoui H, Bourret E, et al. Evaluation of some biological parameters of *Opuntia ficus indica*. 2. Influence of seed supplemented diet on rats. *Bioresour Technol*, 2006 Nov;97(16):2136–40.

Eu CH, Lim WY, Ton SH, et al. Glycyrrhizic acid improved lipoprotein lipase expression, insulin sensitivity, serum lipid and lipid deposition in high-fat diet-induced obese rats. *Lipids Health Dis*, 2010 Jul 29; 9:81.

Ferreira EB, de Assis Rocha Neves F, da Costa MA, et al. Comparative effects of *Stevia rebaudiana* leaves and stevioside on glycaemia and hepatic gluconeogenesis. *Planta Med*, 2006 Jun;72(8):691–96.

Fulghesu AM, Ciampelli M, Muzj G, et al. N-acetyl-cysteine treatment improves insulin sensitivity in women with polycystic ovary syndrome. *Fertil Steril*, 2002 Jun;77(6):1128–35.

Ganmaa D, Cui X, Feskanich D, et al. Milk, dairy intake and risk of endometrial cancer: A 26-year follow-up. *Int J Cancer*, 2011 Jun 29. doi: 10.1002/ijc.26265.

Gao T, You Q. The study of *Fagopyrum tataricum* complex prescription on type II diabetes rats. *Zhong Yao Cai*, 2001 Jun;24(6):424–26.

Genazzani AD, Lanzoni C, Ricchieri F, et al. Myo-inositol administration positively affects hyperinsulinemia and hormonal parameters in overweight patients with polycystic ovary syndrome. *Gynecol Endocrinol*, 2008 Mar;24(3):139–44.

Goyal SK, Samsher, Goyal RK. Stevia (*Stevia rebaudiana*) a bio-sweetener: A review. *Int J Food Sci Nutr*, 2010 Feb;61(1):1–10.

Gray AM, Flatt PR. Pancreatic and extra-pancreatic effects of the traditional anti-diabetic plant, *Medicago sativa* (lucerne). *Br J Nutr*, 1997 Aug;78(2):325–34.

Gude D. Endocrine disruptors: Ubiquitous, yet less known. *Indian J Endocrinol Metab*, 2011 Apr–Jun; 15(2):143–44

Hahm SW, Park J, Son YS. *Opuntia humifusa* stems lower blood glucose and cholesterol levels in streptozotocin-induced diabetic rats. *Nutr Res*, 2011 Jun;31(6): 479–87.

Han S, Wang Z, Chu J, et al. Effects of flavones of buckwheat flower and leaf on insulin resistance and liver PTP1B in type 2 diabetic rats. *Zhongguo Zhong Yao Za Zhi*, 2009 Dec;34(23):3114–18.

Hargrave KM, Azain MJ, Miner JL. Dietary coconut oil increases conjugated linoleic acid-induced body fat loss in mice independent of essential fatty acid deficiency. *Biochim Biophys Acta*, 2005 Oct 15; 1737(1):52–60.

He K, Liu K, Daviglus M, et al. Magnesium intake and incidence of metabolic syndrome among young adults. *Circulation*, 2006 Apr 4;113(13):1675–82.

Herriot A, Whitcroft S, Jeanes Y. An retrospective audit of patients with polycystic ovary syndrome: The effects of a reduced glycaemic load diet. *J Hum Nutr Diet*, 2008 Aug;21(4):337–45.

Hiroshi K, Ryoji K, Kazuo Y, et al. New sweet diterpene glucosides from *Stevia rebaudiana. Phytochemistry*, 1976;15(6):981–83.

Hu Y, Xin HL, Zhang QY, et al. Anti-nociceptive and anti-hyperprolactinemia activities of *Fructus viticis* and its effective fractions and chemical constituents. *Phytomedicine*, 2007 Oct;14(10):668–74.

Huang CN, Chan KC, Lin WT, et al. *Hibiscus sabdariffa* inhibits vascular smooth muscle cell proliferation and migration induced by high glucose — a mechanism involves connective tissue growth factor signals. *J Agric Food Chem*, 2009 Apr 22;57(8):3073–79.

Humphreys L, Costarelli V. Implementation of dietary and general lifestyle advice among women with polycystic ovarian syndrome. *J R Soc Promot Health*, 2008 Jul;128(4):190–95.

Ibañez-Camacho R, Roman-Ramos R. Hypoglycemic effect of *Opuntia* cactus. *Arch Invest Med* (Mex), 1979;10(4):223–30.

Ibrahim N, Shalaby A, Farag R, et al. Gynecological efficacy and chemical investigation of *Vitex agnus-castus* L. fruits growing in Egypt. *Nat Prod Res*, 2008 Apr 15;22(6):537.

Inada M. A 87-year-old woman with mineralocorticoid excess due to 11 beta-HSD2 deficiency. *Nihon Ronen Igakkai Zasshi*, 2007 Jul;44(4):513–16.

Iuorno MJ, Jakubowicz DJ, Baillargeon JP, et al. Effects of D-chiro-inositol in lean women with the polycystic ovary syndrome. *Endocr Pract*, 2002 Nov–Dec;8(6):417–23.

Jarvi A, Karlstrom B, Granfeldt YE, et al. Improved glycemic control and lipid profile and normalized fibrinolytic activity on a low-glycemic index diet in type 2 diabetic patients. *Diabetes Care*, 1999 Jan;22(1):10–18.

Jeanes YM, Barr S, Smith K, Hart KH. Dietary management of women with polycystic ovary syndrome in the United Kingdom: The role of dietitians. *J Hum Nutr Diet*, 2009 Dec;22(6):551–8.

Jenkins D, Wolever T, Bacon S. Diabetic diets: High carbohydrate combined with high fiber. *Am J Clin Nutr*, 1980 Aug;33(8):1729–33.

Jeppesen PB, Gregersen S, Rolfsen SE. Kakizaki rat. *Metabolism*, 2003 Mar;52(3):372–78.

Josephs RA, Guinn JS, Harper ML, et al. Liquorice consumption and salivary testosterone concentrations. *Lancet*, 2001 Nov 10;358(9293):1613–14.

Jung F, Morowietz C, Kiesewetter H, et al. Effect of *Ginkgo biloba* on fluidity of blood and peripheral microcirculation in volunteers. *Arzneimittelforschung*, 1990 May;40(5):589–93.

Kadar A, Robert L, Miskulin M, et al. Influence of anthocyanoside treatment on the cholesterol-induced atherosclerosis in the rabbit. *Paroi Arterielle*, 1979 Dec;5(4):187–205.

Kalgaonkar S, Almario RU, Gurusinghe D, et al. Differential effects of walnuts vs. almonds on improving metabolic and endocrine parameters in PCOS. *Eur J Clin Nutr*, 2011 Mar;65(3):386–93.

Kannappan S, Anuradha CV. Insulin sensitizing actions of fenugreek seed polyphenols, quercetin & metformin in a rat model. *Indian J Med Res*, 2009 Apr;129(4):401–8.

Kao ES, Tseng TH, Lee HJ, et al. Anthocyanin extracted from *Hibiscus attenuate* oxidized LDL-mediated foam cell formation involving regulation of CD36 gene. *Chem Biol Interact*, 2009 May 15;179(2–3):212–18.

Kapusta I, Stochmal A, Perrone A, et al. Triterpene saponins from barrel medic (*Medicago truncatula*) aerial parts. *J Agric Food Chem*, 2005 Mar 23; 53(6):2164–70.

Kataya H, Hamza A, Ramadan G, et al. Effect of licorice extract on the complications of diabetes nephropathy in rats. *Drug Chem Toxicol*, 2011 Apr;34(2):101–18.

Ko BS, Jang JS, Hong SM, et al. Changes in components, glycyrrhizin and glycyrrhetinic acid, in raw *Glycyrrhiza uralensis* Fisch, modify insulin sensitizing and insulinotropic actions. *Biosci Biotechnol Biochem*, 2007 Jun;71(6):1452–61.

Kochikuzhyil B, Devi K, Fattepur S. Effect of saturated fatty acid-rich dietary vegetable oils on lipid profile, antioxidant enzymes and glucose tolerance in diabetic rats. *Indian J Pharmacol*, 2010 Jun;42(3):142–45.

Kujur R, Singh V, Ram M, et al. Antidiabetic activity and phytochemical screening of crude extract of *Stevia rebaudiana* in alloxan-induced diabetic rats. *Pharmacognosy Res*, 2010 Jul;2(4):258–63.

Kurzer M, Xu X. Dietary phytoestrogens. *Annu Rev Nutr*, 1997;17:353–81.

Lee I, Chan Y, Lin C, et al. Effect of cranberry extracts on lipid profiles in subjects with type 2 diabetes. *Diabet Med*, 2008 Dec;25(12):1473–77.

Lehtonen H, Suomela J, Tahvonen R, et al. Different berries and berry fractions have various but slightly positive effects on the associated variables of metabolic diseases on overweight and obese women. *Eur J Clin Nutr*, 2011 Mar;65(3):394–401.

Levtchenko EN, Deinum J, Knoers NV, et al. From gene to disease: "Apparent mineralocorticoid excess" syndrome, a syndrome with an apparent excess of mineral corticoids. *Ned Tijdschr Geneeskd*, 2007 Mar 24;151(12):692–94.

Li X, Yan H, Wang J. Extract of *Ginkgo biloba* and alpha-lipoic acid attenuate advanced glycation end products accumulation and RAGE expression in diabetic nephropathy rats. *Zhongguo Zhong Xi Yi Jie He Za Zhi*, 2011 Apr;31(4):525–31.

Lim S, Zoellner J, Lee J, et al. Obesity and sugar-sweetened beverages in African-American preschool children: A longitudinal study. *Obesity* (Silver Spring), 2009 Jun;17(6):1262–68.

Linarès E, Thimonier C, Degre M. The effect of NeOpuntia on blood lipid parameters — risk factors for the metabolic syndrome (syndrome X). *Adv Ther*, 2007 Sep–Oct;24(5):1115–25.

Liu M, Wu K, Mao X, et al. Astragalus polysaccharide improves insulin sensitivity in KK-Ay mice: Regulation of PKB/GLUT4 signaling in skeletal muscle. *J Ethnopharmacol*, 2010 Jan 8;127(1):32–37.

Losso J, Holliday D, Finley J, et al. Fenugreek bread: A treatment for diabetes mellitus. *J Med Food*, 2009 Oct;12(5):1046–49.

Lu FR, Shen L, Qin Y, et al. Clinical observation on *Trigonella foenum-graecum* L. total saponins in combination with sulfonylureas in the treatment of type 2 diabetes mellitus. *Chin J Integr Med*, 2008 Mar;14(1):56–60.

Mae T, Kishida H, Nishiyama T, et al. A licorice ethanolic extract with peroxisome proliferator-activated receptor-gamma ligand-binding activity affects diabetes in KK-Ay mice, abdominal obesity in diet-induced obese C57BL mice and hypertension in spontaneously hypertensive rats. *J Nutr*, 2003 Nov;133(11):3369–77.

Maghrani M, Zeggwagh NA, Michel J, et al. Antihypertensive effect of *Lepidium sativum* L. in spontaneously hypertensive rats. *J Ethnopharmacol*, 2005 Aug 22;100(1–2):193–97.

Marles RJ, Farnsworth NR. Antidiabetic plants and their active constituents. *Phytomedicine*, 1995 Oct;2(2):137–89.

Marx-Stoelting P, Pfeil R, Solecki R, et al. Assessment strategies and decision criteria for pesticides with endocrine disrupting properties relevant to humans. *Reprod Toxicol*, 2011 May;31(4):574–84.

Masha A, Manieri C, Dinatale S, et al. Prolonged treatment with N-acetylcysteine and L-arginine restores gonadal function in patients with polycystic ovary syndrome. *J Endocrinol Invest*, 2009 Dec;32(11):870–72.

Mashayekh A, Pham DL, Yousem DM, et al. Effects of *Ginkgo biloba* on cerebral blood flow assessed by quantitative MR perfusion imaging: A pilot study. *Neuroradiology*, 2011 Mar;53(3):185–91.

Mateen AA, Rani PU, Naidu MU, et al. Pharmacodynamic interaction study of *Allium sativum* (garlic) with cilostazol in patients with type II diabetes mellitus. *Indian J Pharmacol*, 2011 May;43(3):270–74.

Matsunaga N, Imai S, Inokuchi Y, et al. Bilberry and its main constituents have neuroprotective effects against retinal neuronal damage in vitro and in vivo. *Mol Nutr Food Res*, 2009 Jul;53(7):869–77.

Miettinen HE, Piippo K, Hannila-Handelberg T, et al. Licorice-induced hypertension and common variants of genes regulating renal sodium reabsorption. *Ann Med*, 2010 Sep;42(6):465–74.

Mikulic Petkovsek M, Slatnar A, Stampar F, Veberic R. The influence of organic/integrated production on the content of phenolic compounds in apple leaves and fruits in four different varieties over a 2-year period. *J Sci Food Agric*, 2010 Nov;90(14):2366–78.

Misra H, Soni M, Silawat N, et al. Antidiabetic activity of medium-polar extract from the leaves of *Stevia rebaudiana* Bert. (Bertoni) on alloxan-induced diabetic rats. *J Pharm Bioallied Sci*, 2011 Apr;3(2):242–48.

Mooren FC, Krüger K, Völker K, et al. Oral magnesium supplementation reduces insulin resistance in non-diabetic subjects: A double-blind, placebo-controlled, randomized trial. *Diabetes Obes Metab*, 2011 Mar; 13(3):281–84.

Moorthy R, Prabhu KM, Murthy PS. Anti-hyperglycemic compound (GII) from fenugreek (*Trigonella foenum-graecum* Linn.) seeds, its purification and effect in diabetes mellitus. *Indian J Exp Biol*, 2010 Nov;48(11):1111–18.

Mozaffari-Khosravi H, Jalali-Khanabadi BA, Afkhami-Ardekani M, et al. Effects of sour tea (*Hibiscus sabdariffa*) on lipid profile and lipoproteins in patients with type II diabetes. *J Altern Complement Med*, 2009 Aug;15(8):899–903.

Muneyyirci-Delale O, Nacharaju VL, Dalloul M, et al. Divalent cations in women with PCOS: implications for cardiovascular disease. *Gynecol Endocrinol*, 2001 Jun;15(3):198–201.

Nakagawa K, Kishida H, Arai N, et al. Licorice flavonoids suppress abdominal fat accumulation and increase in blood glucose level in obese diabetic KK-A(y) mice. *Biol Pharm Bull*, 2004 Nov;27(11):1775–78.

Nascimento NR, Lessa LM, Kerntopf MR, et al. Inositols prevent and reverse endothelial dysfunction in diabetic rat and rabbit vasculature metabolically and by scavenging superoxide. *Proc Natl Acad Sci USA*, 2006 Jan 3;103(1):218–23.

Nasr A. Effect of N-acetyl-cysteine after ovarian drilling in clomiphene citrate-resistant PCOS women: A pilot study. *Reprod Biomed Online*, 2010 Mar;20(3):403–09.

Nasri S, Oryan S, Rohani A, et al. The effects of *Vitex agnus-castus* extract and its interaction with dopaminergic system on LH and testosterone in male mice. *Pak J Biol Sci*, 2007 Jul 15;10(14): 2300–307.

Negro R, Greco G, Mangieri T, et al. The influence of selenium supplementation on postpartum thyroid status in pregnant women with thyroid peroxidase autoantibodies. *J Clin Endocrinol Metab*, 2007 Apr; 92(4):1263–68.

Nishiyama S, Mikeda T, Okada T, et al. Transient hypothyroidism or persistent hyperthyrotropinemia in neonates born to mothers with excessive iodine intake. *Thyroid*, 2004 Dec;14(12):1077–83.

Nunlee-Bland G, Gambhir K, Abrams C, et al. Vitamin D deficiency and insulin resistance in obese African-American adolescents. *J Pediatr Endocrinol Metab*, 2011;24(1–2):29–33.

Oh PS, Lim KT. Glycoprotein (90 kDa) isolated from *Opuntia ficus-indica* var. saboten MAKINO lowers plasma lipid level through scavenging of intracellular radicals in Triton WR-1339-induced mice. *Biol Pharm Bull*, 2006 Jul;29(7):1391–96.

Opsomer G, Wensing T, Laevens H, et al. Insulin resistance: The link between metabolic disorders and cystic ovarian disease in high yielding dairy cows? *Anim Reprod Sci*, 1999 Aug 16;56(3–4):211–22.

Padiya R, Khatua T, Bagul P, et al. Garlic improves insulin sensitivity and associated metabolic syndromes in fructose fed rats. *Nutr Metab* (Lond), 2011 Jul 27; 8(1):53.

Pan A, Sun J, Chen Y, et al. Effects of a flaxseed-derived lignan supplement in type 2 diabetic patients: A randomized, double-blind, cross-over trial. *PLoS One*, 2007 Nov 7;2(11):e1148.

Papaleo E, Unfer V, Baillargeon JP, et al. Contribution of myo-inositol to reproduction. *Eur J Obstet Gynecol Reprod Biol*, 2009 Dec;147(2):120–23.

Park JE, Cha YS. *Stevia rebaudiana* Bertoni extract supplementation improves lipid and carnitine profiles in C57BL/6J mice fed a high-fat diet. *J Sci Food Agric*, 2010 May;90(7):1099–105.

Peterson J, Dwyer J, Adlercreutz H, et al. Dietary lignans: Physiology and potential for cardiovascular disease risk reduction. *Nutr Rev*, 2010 Oct;68(10):571–603.

Public Health Committee of the American Thyroid Association. Iodine supplementation for pregnancy and lactation — United States and Canada: Recommendations of the American Thyroid Association. *Thyroid*, 2006;16(10):949–951.

Racek J. Chromium as an essential element. *Cas Lek Cesk*, 2003;142(6):335–59.

Raffone E, Rizzo P, Benedetto V. Insulin sensitiser agents alone and in co-treatment with r-FSH for ovulation induction in PCOS women. *Gynecol Endocrinol*, 2010 Apr;26(4):275–80.

Rayalam S, Yang J, Della-Fera M, et al. Anti-obesity effects of xanthohumol plus guggulsterone in 3T3-L1 adipocytes. *J Med Food*, 2009 Aug;12(4):846–53.

Reid S, Middleton P, Cossich M, et al. Interventions for clinical and subclinical hypothyroidism in pregnancy. *Cochrane Database Syst Rev*, 2010 Jul 7;(7):CD007752.

Rizk A, Bedaiwy M, Al-Inany H. N-acetyl-cysteine is a novel adjuvant to clomiphene citrate in clomiphene citrate-resistant patients with polycystic ovary syndrome. *Fertil Steril*, 2005 Feb;83(2):367–70.

Schneider B. *Ginkgo biloba* extract in peripheral arterial diseases: Meta-analysis of controlled clinical studies. *Arzneimittelforschung*, 1992 Apr;42(4):428–36.

Sharifi F, Mazloomi S, Hajihosseini R, Mazloomzadeh S. Serum magnesium concentrations in polycystic ovary syndrome and its association with insulin resistance. *Gynecol Endocrinol*, 2012 Jan;28(1):7–11.

Sharma B, Salunke R, Srivastava S, et al. Effects of guggulsterone isolated from *Commiphora mukul* in high fat diet induced diabetic rats. *Food Chem Toxicol*, 2009 Oct;47(10):2631–39.

Shenkin J, Heller K, Warren J, et al. Soft drink consumption and caries risk in children and adolescents. *Gen Dent*, 2003 Jan–Feb;51(1):30–36.

Shi J, Arunasalam K, Yeung D, et al. Saponins from edible legumes: Chemistry, processing, and health benefits. *J Med Food*, 2004 Spring;7(1):67–78.

Simonoff M, Shapcott D, Alameddine S, et al. The isolation of glucose tolerance factors from brewer's yeast and their relation to chromium. *Biol Trace Elem Res*, 1992 Jan–Mar;32:25–38.

Simpson HC, Simpson RW, Lousley S, et al. A high carbohydrate leguminous fiber diet improves all aspects of diabetic control. *Lancet*, 1981 Jan 3; 1(8210):1–5.

Sliutz G, Speiser P, Schultz AM, et al. *Agnus-castus* extracts inhibit prolactin secretion of rat pituitary cells. *Horm Metab Res*, 1993 May;25(5):253–55.

Smyth PP. Role of iodine in antioxidant defence in thyroid and breast disease. *Biofactors*, 2003;19(3–4): 121–30.

Soejarto DD, Compadre CM, Medon PJ, et al. Potential sweetening agents of plant origin. II. Field search for sweet-tasting *Stevia* species. *Economic Botany*, 1983 Jan–Mar; 37(1):71–79.

Søltoft M, Nielsen J, Holst Laursen K, et al. Effects of organic and conventional growth systems on the content of flavonoids in onions and phenolic acids in carrots and potatoes. *J Agric Food Chem*, 2010 Oct 13;58(19):10323–29.

Speth P, Jansen J, Lamers C. Effect of acarbose, pectin, a combination of acarbose with pectin, and placebo on postprandial reactive hypoglycaemia after gastric surgery. *Gut*, 1983 Sep;24(9):798–802.

Stanek M, Borman S, Molskness T, et al. Insulin and insulin-like growth factor stimulation of vascular endothelial growth factor production by luteinized granulosa cells: Comparison between polycystic ovarian syndrome (PCOS) and non-PCOS women. *J Clin Endocrinol Metab*, 2007 Jul;92(7):2726–33.

Stewart PM. Tissue-specific Cushing's syndrome, 11beta-hydroxysteroid dehydrogenases and the redefinition of corticosteroid hormone action. *Eur J Endocrinol*, 2003 Sep;149(3):163–68.

Stoclet JC, Schini-Kerth V. Dietary flavonoids and human health. *Ann Pharm Fr*, 2011 Mar;69(2):78–90.

Takahashi K, Yoshino K, Shirai T, et al. Effect of a traditional herbal medicine (shakuyaku-kanzo-to) on testosterone secretion in patients with polycystic ovary syndrome detected by ultrasound. *Nippon Sanka Fujinka Gakkai Zasshi*, 1988 Jun; 40(6):789–92.

Takeuchi T, Nishii O, Okamura T, et al. Effect of traditional herbal medicine, shakuyaku-kanzo-to, on total and free serum testosterone levels. *Am J Chin Med*, 1989;17(1–2):35–44.

Takikawa M, Inoue S, Horio F, et al. Dietary anthocyanin-rich bilberry extract ameliorates hyperglycemia and insulin sensitivity via activation of AMP-activated protein kinase in diabetic mice. *J Nutr*, 2010 Mar; 140(3):527–33.

Tamagno G. Are changes of prolactin levels the effectors of *Vitex agnus-castus* beneficial effects on the pre-menstrual syndrome? *Maturitas*, 2009 Aug 20;63(4):369.

Tanaka T. A novel anti-dysmenorrhea therapy with cyclic administration of two Japanese herbal medicines. *Clin Exp Obstet Gynecol*, 2003;30(2–3): 95–8.

Tao M, McDowell MA, Saydah SH, et al. Relationship of polyunsaturated fatty acid intake to peripheral neuropathy among adults with diabetes in the National Health and Nutrition Examination Survey (NHANES) 1999. *Diabetes Care*, 2008 Jan;31(1):93–95.

Thomson RL, Buckley JD, Noakes M, et al. The effect of a hypocaloric diet with and without exercise training on body composition, cardiometabolic risk profile, and reproductive function in overweight and obese women with polycystic ovary syndrome. *J Clin Endocrinol Metab*, 2008 Sep;93(9):3373–80.

Ulbricht C, Isaac R, Milkin T, et al. An evidence-based systematic review of stevia by the Natural Standard Research Collaboration. *Cardiovasc Hematol Agents Med Chem*, 2010 Apr;8(2):113–27.

Unfer V, Carlomagno G, Rizzo P, et al. Myo-inositol rather than D-chiro-inositol is able to improve oocyte quality in intracytoplasmic sperm injection cycles: A prospective, controlled, randomized trial. *Eur Rev Med Pharmacol Sci*, 2011 Apr;15(4):452–57.

Urumow T, Wieland OH. On the nature of the glucose tolerance factor from yeast. *Horm Metab Res*, 1984 Dec;16 Suppl 1:51–54.

Vacher P, Prevarskaya N, Skryma R, et al. The lipidosterolic extract from *Serenoa repens* interferes with prolactin receptor signal transduction. *J Biomed Sci*, 1995 Oct;2(4):357–65.

Valentová K, Stejskal D, Bartek J, et al. Maca (*Lepidium meyenii*) and yacon (*Smallanthus sonchifolius*) in combination with silymarin as food supplements: In vivo safety assessment. *Food Chem Toxicol*, 2008 Mar;46(3):1006–13.

Vandenberg LN, Chahoud I, Heindel JJ, et al. Urinary, circulating, and tissue biomonitoring studies indicate widespread exposure to bisphenol A. *Environ Health Perspect*, 2010 Aug; 118(8): 1055–70.

van Uum SH, Lenders JW, Hermus AR. Cortisol, 11beta-hydroxysteroid dehydrogenases, and hypertension. *Semin Vasc Med*, 2004 May; 4(2):121–28.

Vecera R, Orolin J, Skottová N, et al. The influence of maca (*Lepidium meyenii*) on antioxidant status, lipid and glucose metabolism in rats. *Plant Foods Hum Nutr*, 2007 Jun;62(2):59–63.

Vincent JB. Recent advances in the nutritional biochemistry of trivalent chromium. *Proc Nutr Soc*, 2004 Feb;63(1):41–47.

Webster DE, He Y, Chen SN, et al. Opioidergic mechanisms underlying the actions of *Vitex agnus-castus* L. *Biochem Pharmacol*, 2011 Jan 1; 81(1):170–77.

Westphal L, Polan M, Trant A. Double-blind, placebo-controlled study of Fertilityblend: A nutritional supplement for improving fertility in women. *Clin Exp Obstet Gynecol*, 2006;33(4):205–08.

Wu X, Yang Y, Huang D. Effect of aqueous extract of *Lepidium apetalum* on dog's left ventricular function. *Zhong Yao Cai*, 1998 May;21(5):243–45.

Wu Y, Li S, Cui W, et al. *Ginkgo biloba* extract improves coronary blood flow in healthy elderly adults: Role of endothelium-dependent vasodilation. *Phytomedicine*, 2008 Mar;15(3):164–69.

Wu Y, Li S, Zu X, et al. *Ginkgo biloba* extract improves coronary artery circulation in patients with coronary artery disease: Contribution of plasma nitric oxide and endothelin–1. *Phytother Res*, 2008 Jun;22(6):734–39.

Wuttke W, Jarry H, Christoffel V, et al. Chaste tree (*Vitex agnus-castus*) — pharmacology and clinical indications. *Phytomedicine*, 2003 May;10(4):348–57.

Xu LZ, Li R, Sun ZJ, et al. The relationship between leptin, insulin-like growth factor-1 (IGF-1) and hyperinsulinemia of patients with polycystic ovarian syndrome. *Sichuan Da Xue Xue Bao Yi Xue Ban*, 2006 Nov;37(6):882–85.

Xu ME, Xiao SZ, Sun YH, et al. Effects of astragaloside IV on pathogenesis of metabolic syndrome in vitro. *Acta Pharmacol Sin*, 2006 Feb;27(2):229–36.

Yao N, Lan F, He RR, et al. Protective effects of bilberry (*Vaccinium myrtillus* L.) extract against endotoxin-induced uveitis in mice. *J Agric Food Chem*, 2010 Apr 28;58(8):4731–36.

Yin J, Xing H, Ye J. Efficacy of berberine in patients with type 2 diabetes mellitus. *Metabolism*, 2008 May;57(5):712–17.

Yin X, Zhang Y, Yu J, et al. The antioxidative effects of astragalus saponin I protect against development of early diabetic nephropathy. *J Pharmacol Sci*, 2006 Jun;101(2):166–73.

Yuan HN, Wang CY, Sze CW, et al. A randomized, crossover comparison of herbal medicine and bromocriptine against risperidone-induced hyperprolactinemia in patients with schizophrenia. *J Clin Psychopharmacol*, 2008 Jun;28(3):264–370.

Zamansoltani F, Nassiri-Asl M, Sarookhani MR, et al. Antiandrogenic activities of *Glycyrrhiza glabra* in male rats. *Int J Androl*, 2009 Aug;32(4):417–22.

Zhang H, Wei J, Xue R, et al. Berberine lowers blood glucose in type 2 diabetes mellitus patients through increasing insulin receptor expression. *Metabolism*, 2010 Feb;59(2):285–92.

Zhang HW, Zhang YH, Lu MJ, et al. Comparison of hypertension, dyslipidaemia and hyperglycaemia between buckwheat seed-consuming and non-consuming Mongolian-Chinese populations in Inner Mongolia, China. *Clin Exp Pharmacol Physiol*, 2007 Sep;34(9):838–44.

Zhang N, Wang XH, Mao SL, et al. Astragaloside IV improves metabolic syndrome and endothelium dysfunction in fructose-fed rats. *Molecules*, 2011 May 10;16(5):3896–907.

Zhang W, Wang X, Liu Y, et al. Dietary flaxseed lignan extract lowers plasma cholesterol and glucose concentrations in hypercholesterolaemic subjects. *Br J Nutr*, 2008 Jun;99(6):1301–9.

Zhong G, Chen B. Serum and follicular fluid levels of IGF-II, IGF-binding protein-4 and pregnancy-associated plasma protein-A in controlled ovarian hyperstimulation cycle between polycystic ovarian syndrome (PCOS) and non-PCOS women. *Gynecol Endocrinol*, 2011 Feb;27(2):86–90.

Zhou J, Zhou S. Berberine regulates peroxisome proliferator-activated receptors and positive transcription elongation factor b expression in diabetic adipocytes. *Eur J Pharmacol*, 2010 Dec 15; 649(1–3):390–97.

Zimmermann M, Delange F. Iodine supplementation of pregnant women in Europe: a review and recommendations. *Eur J Clin Nutr*, 2004 Jul;58(7): 979–84.

Zimmermann MB. Iodine deficiency in pregnancy and the effects of maternal iodine supplementation on the offspring: A review. *Am J Clin Nutr*, 2009 Feb;89(2):668S–72S.

Zou F, Mao XQ, Wang N, et al. Astragalus polysaccharides alleviates glucose toxicity and restores glucose homeostasis in diabetic states via activation of AMPK. *Acta Pharmacol Sin*, 2009 Dec;30(12):1607–15.

Contributing Authors

Byron Ayanoglu
125 Best Vegetarian Recipes
A recipe from this book appears on page 230.

Johanna Burkhard
Diabetes Comfort Food
Recipes from this book appear on pages 158, 164, 165 and 222.

Dietitians of Canada
Cook!
Recipes from this book appear on pages 163, 168, 169, 171, 173, 174, 177, 179, 180, 186, 188, 191, 193, 200, 203, 216 and 217.

Dietitians of Canada
Cook Great Food
Recipes from this book appear on pages 162, 166 (top), 170, 178, 189, 192, 196–198, 202, 204, 206–212, 214, 215, 218, 223, 225–228, 231 and 232.

Dietitians of Canada
Simply Great Food
Recipes from this book appear on pages 156, 157, 166 (bottom), 167, 172, 176, 181–185, 190, 194, 195, 199, 201, 213, 219, 220, 224, 229 and 233–236.

Camilla Saulsbury
5 Easy Steps to Healthy Cooking
Recipes from this book appear on pages 239–241, 243 and 244.

Donna Washburn and Heather Butt
250 Gluten-Free Favorites
Recipes from this book appear on pages 159–161.

Library and Archives Canada Cataloguing in Publication

Stansbury, Jill
    The PCOS health & nutrition guide : includes 125 recipes for managing Polycystic Ovarian Syndrome / Jillian Stansbury with Sheila Mitchell.

Includes index.
ISBN 978-0-7788-0405-5

    1. Polycystic ovary syndrome—Popular works. 2. Polycystic ovary syndrome—Diet therapy—Recipes. 3. Polycystic ovary syndrome—Nutritional aspects. I. Mitchell, Sheila II. Title.

RG480.S7S83 2012   618.1'10654   C2011-907496-6

Index